LIZ EARLE'S
QUICK GUIDES
Cod Liver Oil

LIZ EARLE'S
QUICK GUIDES
Cod Liver Oil

BⓉXTREE

Advice to the Reader

Before following any advice contained in this book, it is recommended that you consult your doctor if you suffer from any health problems or special condition or are in any doubt.

First published in Great Britain in 1995 by Boxtree Limited, Broadwall House, 21 Broadwall, London SE1 9PL

The right of Liz Earle to be identified as Author of this Work has been asserted by her in accordance with the Copyright, Designs and Patents Act 1988

10 9 8 7 6 5 4 3 2

ISBN: 0 7522 1641 4

Text design by Blackjacks
Cover design by Hammond Hammond

Printed and Bound in Great Britain by Cox & Wyman Ltd, Reading, Berkshire

A CIP catalogue entry for this book is available from the British Library

Contents

Acknowledgements 6

Introduction 7

1 The History of Cod Liver Oil 9

2 Cod Liver Oil Science 19

3 The Link with Arthritis 35

4 Common Skin Disorders 45

5 Future Benefits 59

6 The Oily Fish Diet 71

Glossary 83

Useful Addresses 87

Index 89

ACKNOWLEDGEMENTS

I am grateful to Sheila Lavery for helping to produce this book. I would also like to thank Dr Ray Rice of The Fish Foundation and food historian Jennifer Stead. My gratitude also to Beverley Banson, Liz Griffith and all at Seven Seas for access to valuable research material. I am indebted to the talented team at Boxtree, Rosemary Sandberg and Claire Bowles Publicity for their unfailing enthusiasm and support.

Introduction

Cod liver oil is the single best-selling supplement in the British Isles. Many millions have benefited from their daily spoonful, although not as many know exactly why this golden liquid is so beneficial. Cod liver oil is not a magical elixir. It contains certain nutrients which have been well-researched by the scientific and medical professions. After many hundreds of years of use, modern day analysis means we can now understand how cod liver oil can help many severe ailments, including arthritis, psoriasis and heart disease. This *Quick Guide* reveals all you need to know about this fascinating food supplement and its many benefits.

Liz Earle

—1—
The History of Cod Liver Oil

If you thought that cod liver oil disappeared with the hand-knitted socks of post-war Britain, it's time to think again. Cod liver oil is still the biggest selling supplement in Britain. Faithful followers are convinced that its nutritional benefits far outweigh those of the synthetic vitamins that stock the shelves of chemists and healthfood stores, and now it seems that science supports this belief. An increasing amount of research credits cod liver oil with benefiting everything from dry skin to heart disease and premature birth, and a whole new generation of Britons has become cod liver oil conscious.

Who would have imagined that a product of such humble origins could play such a vital role in the health of a nation? Before it was accepted as a food supplement or remedy, cod liver oil had been used for centuries by the poor of the north of England, Scotland, Ireland, northern Europe, Iceland and Newfoundland to fuel their lamps, soften leather and make textiles. It was also used in animal feed. Perhaps the resulting glossy coats and healthy constitution of their animals encouraged people to take it themselves.

In fishing communities, its role as a medicine predates other uses. The fishermen of Shetland used to rub it on aching joints and troublesome skin conditions. It was absorbed through the skin, but very slowly, and people probably thought they would get faster results from drinking it.

In original form, the oil was treacle black and foul smelling – a less appetising brew you could scarcely imagine. It was a brave soul who bridged that gap between smelly muscular rub and vile tonic.

Folklore records how Iceland's poor used to eat fish liver oils mixed with mutton tallow. The combination, known as '*broedingur*' was one of the earliest recorded healthfoods. Closer to home, Shetlanders are known to have feasted on such appetising delights as 'krappin and stap' – fish liver and oatmeal stuffed into a large fish head or made into a dumpling. Another Shetland speciality was 'cod liver bannock' – cod livers mixed with oatmeal, soda, salt and pepper, and boiled. A bannock was so nutrient-packed it could keep you going for twenty-four hours and Shetlanders believed 'It gives our young men supple backs, it gives our lasses sap.'

Shetlanders in general were partial to a drop of the fishy stuff. To fight colds when out at sea some fishermen are reputed to have popped a couple of raw livers between two slices of bread and let the skipper sit on it while he steered the boat. The result: bread soaked in freshly squeezed fish oil.

Elsewhere in Britain folk weren't quite so brave. Records show that eighteenth-century Norfolk was also enlightened about the benefits of fish oil, but drinking it was out of the question. In the *Diary of a Country Parson*, the Rev. James Woodforde (1758–81) recorded that:

> *Mr Thorne sent Nancy over today some Cod's liver oil about a Quarter of a Pint, for her to make use of about her stiff arm and lame knee – she began it this evening on her arm only – Pray God! Send thy blessing upon it for her good.*

Even today, older people, who may have been rubbed with cod liver oil as children, still use it on their joints and on scars that won't heal. In the latter case, it apparently still works wonders.

A friend was anxious about an operation scar that wouldn't heal. His elderly neighbour recommended he rub cod liver oil on it – and it worked.

In Nigeria cod liver oil has acquired an almost religious significance. In a ritual, mothers rub it like a magic potion on to the fontanelle of their newborn baby. This helps to close the fontanelle. After this happens, the oil is rubbed into the rest of the body to bring a healthy glow to the skin. But, according to superstition, it mustn't touch the head. If it does, the baby's head is said to grow much larger than the rest of the body!

Cod Liver Oil as Medicine

Cod liver oil enjoyed centuries of fame as a folk medicine before it received any medical backing. The earliest records of its medical use in England date back to February 1782, when a certain Dr Darbey and Dr Samuel Kay, a physician at the Manchester Royal Infirmary, made the first recorded clinical trial. They claimed that, ten years earlier, they had discovered 'by accident' that cod liver oil was successful in cases of chronic rheumatism, 'but it is little known in any county except Lancashire.' Down in Norfolk the Rev. James Woodforde would no doubt have disagreed.

Rheumatism was a sort of catch-all term for diseased or aching limbs or joints. It was widely known even before Darbey and Kay's study showed that cod liver oil was an effective treatment for bone diseases and rheumatic conditions, but no one knew how or why it worked. Doctors and patients alike genuinely believed that it worked by oiling the joints – a myth that prevailed for many years.

Such was the effect of cod liver oil on rheumatic conditions that Dr Kay claimed to dispense between fifty and sixty gallons a year 'for almost every lameness'. He is recorded as saying that,

'Except bark, opium and mercury, I believe no one medicine in the materia medica is likely to be of better service.' Thankfully bark, opium and mercury, are no longer the medicines of the people, but cod liver oil continues to appeal to health-conscious Britons.

Kay and Darbey's work was not immediately followed up in Britain. A German doctor by the name of Schenk did his own research, based on the Manchester findings, and discovered that cod liver oil was also effective against rickets, a crippling bone disease that affected nine out of ten children during the industrial revolution. Rickets occurs in children as a result of vitamin D deficiency – this vitamin is a major ingredient in cod liver oil. This research took place before the discovery of vitamins, so nobody knew why cod liver oil was such an effective cure-all. These early trials merely acknowledged its efficacy – its chemical composition was a mystery.

In 1841 in Edinburgh, John Bennett (who had studied in France and Germany) brought out his famous *Oleum Jecoris Aselli*, in which he stated that cod liver oil was being used medicinally in France and Germany but he wasn't aware that it was used much in Britain. After the publication of Bennett's book, doctors started using it to treat consumption and scrofula (tuberculosis of the skin), common diseases exacerbated by malnutrition. Around the same time, a Dutch doctor called Ludovicus Josephus de Jongh produced a book similar to Bennett's. An 1849 English translation stimulated a surge of medical papers in England. Dr de Jongh wrote various papers extolling the benefits of cod liver oil as a 'curative'. After prescribing it for twelve years for a range of illnesses from tuberculosis to sciatica and rheumatism, Dr de Jongh wrote in *The Lancet*:

> *It may be given with confidence in all cases where the powers of life are low and where the improper assimilation of food is the cause. It affords nourishment*

when none can be borne, restores the functions of
digestion, and furnishes the frame with fat in a truly
wonderful manner.

But Dr de Jongh did not favour just any cod liver oil. With the introduction of steam processing in the mid-nineteenth century, the quality and taste of the oil improved and demand for it grew. The consequent boom in trade led to some unscrupulous Dutch suppliers passing off impure concoctions as pure cod liver oil. De Jongh discovered that these evil brews, often adulterated with decayed herring oil and seal fat simply didn't have the healing abilities of pure cod liver oil. He became dedicated to bringing pure cod liver oil to the people, for which he was honoured by the Queen of The Netherlands and commended by Dr Fouquerier, personal physician to King Louis Philippe of France.

De Jongh was an obviously avid cod liver oil fan and a very influential figure in the early medical science of cod liver oil. His clinical work initiated the world-famous experiment on London Zoo lion cubs which were saved from the usual fate of cubs in captivity – death by rickets. Gradually, doctors began to realise the scope of this natural remedy. They also noticed that, for whatever reason, cod liver oil was particularly effective against diseases associated with malnutrition.

Dr de Jongh's research into animals with rickets was backed up in 1923 when Professor Chick, in Vienna, found that cod liver oil was a successful treatment for children with rickets. By this time cod liver oil had received a little extra backing from the scientific world. Vitamin A was recognised in 1913 and cod liver oil was deemed a rich source. Some time later, when vitamin D was identified, cod liver oil was lauded once again. After years of being little more than a rather foul-tasting folk remedy cod liver oil had taken its first steps on the road to nutritional stardom.

Early Production in England

Cod liver oil came into common usage via North Atlantic cod fishermen. When they brought the fish back to shore, they'd gut them and throw the livers into a barrel where they would rot to produce a foul-smelling black oil. Up until 1850, the fishermen of Hull did likewise. But for speed, and to preserve the fish, they gutted their catch at sea and threw the livers into a storage barrel where they fermented for three or four weeks. The Hull fishermen sold this unrefined cod liver oil to the tanning industry and to animal feed manufacturers to supplement their meagre income. But the oil they produced was crude and not suitable for medicinal purposes. At this time the bulk of medicinal cod liver oil was imported from Norway.

In 1850, things started to improve. Just two years earlier a Scarborough man discovered that, instead of being left to rot, the livers would produce a clean-tasting oil when they were heated with steam. The steam method was well under way by 1853. It was popular because it enabled the fishermen to extract more oil of a much higher quality. The oil itself was paler in colour and marginally better in taste. Some people used this refined oil medicinally, but it was still very crude compared to modern standards and most of it was used for animal feed.

In the nineteenth century trawlers could be at sea for three or four weeks at a time. They would travel up to 3,000 miles to the coldest parts of the world to catch cod. Once there, they would fish like fury until they'd caught about ten tons of cod. The fish were gutted, beheaded and stored on ice to keep them fresh. The livers were thrown into barrels. By the time they came home the fisherman would have caught enough fish to produce about 4,000 gallons of cod liver oil. Cod have unusually large livers and it takes just ten livers to produce a gallon of oil. The barrels of livers were taken to the nearby factory where they were steamed. The resulting oil, which was known as cod oil, and some of the better quality stuff, which was called cattle oil, was used for animal feed. However, by the mid-1930s this low-grade oil wasn't even thought fit for livestock.

The 1930s were a turning point for British cod liver oil production. Doctors had eventually accepted that cod liver oil could prevent and cure rickets, and demand for cod liver oil soared. Around the same time, some of the trawler men began to experiment with sea boiling – steaming the livers at sea while they were still fresh. Very soon a trawler docked at Hull with a quantity of sea-boiled oil which was good enough for veterinary use and possibly good enough to be processed to medicinal quality. Gradually, as more and more trawlers became equipped, the production of sea-boiled cod liver oil increased. This all meant extra work for the fishermen. Traditionally, they had made very little money out of the cod liver oil business – it was just a little side-line for them. So, to compensate for their extra workload, owners agreed to pay them what was known as 'liver money'. This was an early example of performance-related pay and each crew were paid in proportion to the amount of oil they brought in.

At this time there were several fishing companies operating out of Hull. However, they agreed that it would be in their best interests to pool their resources instead of working in several small independent operations. So, in June 1934 the British Cod Liver Oil Producers (BCLO) was formed. BCLO (which later became Seven Seas) operated as a co-operative and ploughed money back into the industry and the men who worked in it.

Under the auspices of the BCLO the Hull trawler men produced a variety of wonderful sounding oils: cod oil, pale cod oil, cattle oil, ruby oil and dark cod oil, most of which was being used in industry, with the best going into making animal feed. Eventually, BCLO started to produce a highly refined medicinal oil that conformed to pharmaceutical standards. The company was able to achieve this with the help of a new factory at

Marfleet. It was the world's largest cod liver oil refinery with an expensive array of clarifying, bleaching and deodorising equipment to produce the smooth golden deodorised liquid that the public demanded.

By 1936 the first British-produced medicinal oil was available. Veterinary oil was already being marketed under the name of Solvitax. It may have sounded more like a pack of headache pills than a rich source of natural goodness, but it sold by the gallon. The name for the new medicinal quality oil was to be Seven Seas. Unfortunately for those who didn't like even the new refined taste the concept of capsules was still a long way off. But, fishy taste or not, with the help of King Cod, the company's gigantic promotional fish, by the time of the Second World War the country was awash with cod liver oil.

King Cod Goes to War

The outbreak of the Second World War changed everything in the fishing industry. Trawlers were requisitioned by the Royal Navy and the abundant supplies of cod liver oil began to dwindle.

By this time, the health benefits of cod liver oil were undisputed. The Ministry of Food established the Welfare Foods scheme, which involved the free distribution of cod liver oil to protect against malnutrition in pregnant and breastfeeding mothers, all children under the age of five and people over forty. The oil was sometimes distributed with free concentrated orange juice, or women were advised to give it to their children in milk. Others simply had a spoonful of the stuff, doled out by the firm hand of the school nurse.

To meet this huge demand, oil had to be imported from Iceland and processed at Marfleet. Although this was initially a necessity it led to oil being imported on a regular basis, even after the war ended.

The Government was so delighted with the results of the Welfare Foods scheme that it was decided that the scheme should continue indefinitely. Despite rationing, bombings and hardship, Britain's war babies were the healthiest the nation had ever produced. They were taller, stronger and heavier than pre-war babies and rickets was a thing of the past. The daily spoonful of cod liver oil had paid off and a whole generation of children had become accustomed to its distinctive flavour.

Cod liver oil continued to be distributed free at heath clinics until 1971, when it was stopped because it had become so unpopular. People had become attracted to the tasteless synthetic vitamin pills that were flooding the health market. Cod liver oil was thought of as old-fashioned and something that was forced on you as a child. Of course, by now it was also available in a tasteless capsule form and many people continued to take these. Others stuck with the war-time favourite – cod liver oil mixed with malt. This sticky concoction was also high in B vitamins, but you had to wind it around a spoon to break the treacly thread that would dribble down the side of the jar as well as over your hands and chin. Some children, myself included, found it delicious. It is still available but has since fallen out of favour because of its high calorie content.

In the 1970s the bulk of oil went into the manufacture of animal foods as well as leather and plastic goods, paints and emulsifiers. BCLO had also branched out into producing hydrogenated vegetable oils for baking, frying, confectionery and canning. Meanwhile, in the background, research was unearthing ever-increasing information about the benefits of cod liver oil as a healthfood. King Cod was getting ready to make a comeback.

—— 2 ——

Cod Liver Oil Science

As cod liver oil became increasingly refined and more widely consumed, producers realised the need for scientific research into how and why cod liver oil was beneficial to health. The extensive nineteenth-century work of Dr de Jongh had paved the way for in-depth research.

De Jongh was the first person to attempt an analysis of the chemical composition of cod liver oil. He claimed it included: oleic acid, margaric acid, glycerine, butyric acid, acetic acid, fellinic acid, sulphuric acid, phosphorus, chalk, chalinic acid, bilifulvine, iodine, bromine, chlorine, phosphoric acid, magnesia and soda. He was correct about some of these ingredients, but with others he was completely wrong. Even the ingredients which he accurately pin-pointed, such as oleic acid, were of limited nutritional value except as a source of calories.

Not surprisingly, Dr de Jongh is remembered and respected for his clinical work rather than this analysis, which is now completely redundant. De Jongh's analysis took place before the discovery of vitamins and well before anyone knew about essential fatty acids. So, although it was important in its time, it is hopelessly inadequate by today's standards as it makes no mention of the nutrients which are most important of all, ie vitamins A and D and essential fatty acids (EFAs).

The big breakthrough came in the 1920s when vitamins were discovered and cod liver oil was found to be a rich source of vitamins A and D. Vitamin A is necessary for healthy skin, growth and development. Vitamin D is vital for strong bones. Vitamin D deficiency causes rickets in children, and the disease had blighted the lives of nineteenth-century children, who were often malnourished and spent much of their time working in factories. Long hours in such dark and dreary conditions meant that they rarely felt the sunlight on their skin. Exposure to sunlight is one very important way in which our bodies can make vitamin D.

Once scientists understood the role of vitamins in the body they could see why cod liver oil had been so beneficial for rickets and rheumatism especially, and also for skin diseases such as scrofula.

The Main Ingredients

We've come a long way since de Jongh's analysis, yet despite years of research we still don't have a complete picture of what makes up cod liver oil. It's almost as if the oil is greater than the sum of its parts. We do know however, that it contains at least five important ingredients.

VITAMIN A (RETINOL)

Vitamin A was the first vitamin to be identified, and foods rich in vitamin A were used medicinally as long ago as 1500BC. Cod liver oil is a very rich source of vitamin A, which is sometimes called the skin vitamin as it is needed to repair skin tissues and vitamin A deficiency can lead to spots, acne and dry scaly skin. It is also needed for strong hair and nails, good eyesight and healthy growth in children.

Vitamin A helps to build an efficient immune system and protects against respiratory infections. As a fat-soluble vitamin it is stored in the liver. High levels of vitamin A can be toxic so always stick to the recommended dose of cod liver oil.

VITAMIN D

The high vitamin D content of cod liver oil made it a valuable weapon in the battle against rickets in the nineteenth and early twentieth centuries.

Vitamin D is widely known as 'the sunshine vitamin' because it can be generated in the body by exposing the skin to sunlight. Lack of sunlight combined with malnutrition was the main reason why rickets was so rife among nineteenth-century factory children.

Cod liver oil is still one of the most important natural sources of this essential vitamin, which is necessary for the growth of healthy teeth and bones. Vitamin D does this by helping the body to absorb calcium and phosphorus. It also protects against a bone disease called osteomalacia in adults, and loss of bone (osteoporosis) in later years. Like vitamin A it is fat soluble and can be stored in the liver. So even though we don't get much sunshine during British winters, healthy and safe exposure during the summer can build up the body's reserves. But too much vitamin D can be toxic, and as a natural defence people who live in very hot countries are genetically protected by having darker skin. Unfortunately, when dark-skinned people move to the less sunny climes of northern Europe, they are unlikely to get enough vitamin D.

Asian women and children are particularly vulnerable as they get very little of this important vitamin from their diet and they also tend to cover up when out of doors. Consequently, rickets has resurfaced as a modern problem. In fact in 1983, the Minister of Health launched a rickets prevention campaign among Asian families in Britain.

VITAMIN E

One of the antioxidant nutrients. It protects against free-radicals, the destructive particles that can damage cells and lead to disease. It has been noticed that people who eat a diet rich in vitamin E are better protected against heart disease and some types of cancer.

In fact, vitamin E plays a variety of roles in the body. It improves skin texture, delays ageing, boosts energy levels, strengthens blood vessels and reduces the risk of clotting. It also improves muscle strength and influences hormones. Vitamin E is added to cod liver oil to act as a natural preservative for the omega-3 oils, which are susceptible to oxidation.

ESSENTIAL FATTY ACIDS

Although the vitamin content of cod liver oil is important, it is the essential fatty acid (EFA) content that has excited so much medical and scientific interest.

Essential fatty acids were discovered in 1929 and are so-called because they are essential to the normal healthy functioning of the body. They cannot be made in the body so we have to get them from our food. EFAs are the major building blocks of the fats in us and in the food we eat; they protect our internal organs and are important sources of energy. They also make up the protective membrane that envelops each one of the cells in our body.

Fatty acids can be either monounsaturated or polyunsaturated and consist of a chain of carbon and hydrogen atoms. The length of the chain determines their use in the body. The shortest chains are four carbon atoms long. An example of this length of chain is butyric acid, found in butter. Cod liver oil is an example of a long-chain polyunsaturated fatty acid. It is eighteen carbon atoms long, the same length as EFAs found in brain tissue.

The most important essential fatty acids fall into two families: omega-3s and omega-6s. Omega-3s, derived from alpha-linolenic acid, are richest in fish, but also come from pumpkin seeds, walnuts, flax and soya beans. They are an important but often underestimated part of a healthy diet. The more well-known family is the omega-6s, from linoleic acid. They are found in sunflower, safflower, sesame seeds and, most famously, in evening primrose oil. Most people have a higher intake of omega-6s than omega-3s.

Omega-3s differ in subtle but important ways from the polyunsaturates found in vegetable oils and polyunsaturated margarines. The main omega-3 polyunsaturates are EPA (eicosapentaenoic acid) and DHA (docosahexaenoic acid). They derive from linolenic acid and are used by the body to make prostaglandins and to regulate leukotrienes.

Prostaglandins are complex hormone-like chemicals which regulate cellular activity in the body. There are three families of prostaglandins and the third family have potent anti-clotting properties. Leukotrienes are made from arachidonic acid (AA), the fatty acid found in eggs, red meat and other animal protein. They are important agents which, in the right amounts, protect the body against disease and infection. But too much can cause inflammation. Diseases such as rheumatoid arthritis, MS and asthma are cases where the body seems to react to harmless substances because of high levels of leukotrienes. Counteracting high levels of arachidonic acid with EPA can reduce inflammation.

Both EPA and DHA form part of normal human tissue. They are present in brain cells, the nervous system, retina, inner ear, adrenal and sex glands and low levels of them in the body can cause serious health problems. DHA is the main polyunsaturate in the thinking part of the brain. It is considered necessary for early brain development, which lends scientific weight to the old wives' tale that fish is good for the brain. There is a tremendous surge of DHA in the brain of an unborn child in the last three months of pregnancy.

EPA helps to lower blood fats known as triglycerides and reduces blood clotting. The early research into the Eskimo diet revealed that their high fish consumption meant they had very high levels of EPA in their blood and, not surprisingly, very low rates of coronary heart disease. Its anti-inflammatory properties help to regulate diseases such as rheumatoid arthritis and psoriasis.

The First Clinical Studies

One of the first reports of cod liver oil being used medicinally in this century appeared in the *Archives of International Medicine* in March 1920. Professor Ralph Pemberton of the University of Pennsylvania, wrote of how he had used cod liver oil to treat 400 military patients with arthritis with great success.

Shortly afterwards, in August 1923, a thesis extolling the benefits of cod liver oil in the treatment of rickets, rheumatism, gout and other joint disorders was published in the *American Journal of Diseases of Children*. The author, Ruth Guy, was a doctor in the Department of Pediatrics at Yale University School of Medicine. What she produced was actually a historical treatise and not a set of clinical findings, but her work was long regarded as a landmark thesis in research into the therapeutic value of cod liver oil. The first real scientific paper on cod liver oil investigated the role of this fish oil in the treatment of arthritis. It appeared in a 1959 edition of *The Journal of the National Medicine Association*. This study is described in greater detail in the next chapter.

While this research was going on, sales of medicinal cod liver oil were taking a battering from synthetic vitamin pills. Many people felt that it was easier to take vitamin A and D supplements than to take a spoonful of cod liver oil which, apart from being hard to stomach, also contained more calories. So research continued to see if the oil contained other important nutrients apart from vitamins A and D.

In 1955 a study at the Marfleet biological testing station showed encouraging and rather surprising results about how synthetic versions of vitamins A and D compared with those that occurred naturally in cod liver oil. Three popular chicken-feed mashes containing synthetic forms of vitamins A and D were used to feed 100 chickens ranging in age from one day to eight weeks. The chickens were divided into three groups which were then divided into two sub-groups. One sub-group received a small dose of Solvitax (the veterinary quality cod liver oil) with their mash, while the other did not. At the end of eight weeks there were significant differences between the chickens. Those on cod liver oil were heavier, healthier, better feathered and more mature than the other birds.

This study led to more research into natural versus synthetic vitamins in the treatment of human illnesses. In 1956 Professor Frazer, Head of the Department of Pharmacology at the University of Birmingham, began a detailed research programme into the effects of cod liver oil on tuberculosis sufferers. Synthetic vitamin A was shown to have no effect on the disease at all, but cod liver oil did seem to confer some benefits. Professor Frazer believed that some of cod liver oil's benefits might be due to ingredients other than just vitamins. At his instigation researchers began to investigate more fully the chemical composition of cod liver oil.

The Cholesterol Connection

By this time scientists knew that polyunsaturated oils, which are present in vegetable and cod liver oils, had physiological benefits when taken into the body. International research showed that polyunsaturated oils reduced levels of cholesterol in the blood. Cholesterol has several important roles in normal body functioning. It is used to make hormones and fat cells and to carry vitamins around the body. But even in the 1950s it was known to be a contributory factor in heart disease.

In 1961 *The Lancet* published a paper by Kingsbury, Morgan, Aylott and Emmerson who, in a study at St Mary's Medical

School in London, had found that two tablespoons of cod liver oil a day considerably reduced cholesterol levels in participants.

The Discovery of Omega-3s

At the beginning of the 1970s, Doctors J Dyerberg and HO Bang studied the health of Eskimos in Greenland. They found that Eskimos eat a great deal of fatty fish and seafood such as seal and whale blubber, which is high in cholesterol, yet they have a very low rate of heart disease and practically no incidence of diabetes. However, they also found that when Eskimos moved to Canada and adopted a typically Canadian diet they developed the same rate of heart disease as other Canadians. Dyerberg and Bang concluded that diet had something to do with it.

Indeed it had. Eskimos on a traditional high-fish diet had very high levels of an essential fatty acid called eicosapentaenoic acid (EPA) in their blood. High levels of EPA in the blood means that their blood doesn't clot as quickly as other people's, so they are less likely to suffer from conditions such as heart disease and thrombosis. EPA and docosahexaenoic acid (DHA) make up omega-3 polyunsaturate essential fatty acids, in which cod liver oil is rich.

The findings on omega-3s leant weight to the claim that fish is good for your heart. The world of science agreed that a diet high in omega-3 EFAs could reduce the risk of heart disease. Essential fatty acids also come from other sources. Vegetable oils, corn oil, sesame and sunflower seeds are also high in these and for a long time it was assumed that there was no difference between these and the essential fatty acids found in fish.

Then in 1983 TAB Saunders and Farah Roshanai conducted a further study into the benefits of EPA. They made a controlled crossover comparison of the effects of linseed oil, which is also a source of EPA, and a fish oil-based supplement. The supplement they chose was MaxEPA, which is high in both EPA and DHA but low in vitamins A and D. This allows a high intake of essential fatty acids without the risk of vitamin overdose.

The study was in two parts: first the volunteers added a small amount of linseed oil to their diet for two weeks; then they left a gap of six weeks and did the same with MaxEPA. The participants took 5g, 10g and 20g of MaxEPA a day for three separate three-week periods. The results showed that linseed oil raised levels of EPA in the body only slightly, and much less than MaxEPA, even at 5g a day. MaxEPA had the added benefit of lowering cholesterol levels.

The Benefits in Heart Disease

Coronary heart disease was one of the first areas of medicine to benefit from research into fish oils. The levels of heart disease in Britain and America are among the highest in the world. About two million Britons show signs of the disease and in 1985 it accounted for 47 percent of deaths in America. Any improvement on statistics like these could only be greeted with optimism, especially when the results were as encouraging as those from two of the most significant trials ever conducted into fish oils and heart disease. It is no coincidence that these studies were done in Britain and America.

As we have seen, the Eskimos with their fish-rich diet, suffered far less from heart disease than the British and Americans thanks to the essential fatty acids present in fish oil. To find out how, we must first look at what causes a heart attack. The main cause is a blood clot blocking a coronary artery or one of its main branches. There are a number of major risk factors involved in causing blood clots, of which smoking and high levels of blood cholesterol are considered to be the most important.

Cholesterol on its own is not responsible for heart attacks, what we need to be wary of is low density lipoprotein or LDL. This protein carries cholesterol through the blood to the cells that need it. Cholesterol is a vital chemical for our cells, but we tend to have far more than we actually need. Cholesterol is produced in the liver and then transported to our cells by the LDL. However, if there are too few sites in the body where LDL can stop to unload its cargo of cholesterol, it starts to release the cholesterol in unsuitable areas, such as the lining of the coronary arteries. This dumping of fat can start very early on in life and a high cholesterol diet can soon cause a large build up in our blood. This build up of cholesterol around the lining of an artery reduces the size of the area where blood enters the artery, so that less blood can get through. Smoking can exacerbate this condition by hardening the arteries and so allowing even less blood to pass through the artery to the heart.

Fortunately, the body has its own natural defence mechanism to prevent this build up of cholesterol in the form of high density lipoprotein (or HDL) which is created in the liver. Its main function is to circulate through our blood scavenging any excess cholesterol and returning it to the liver where it can be disposed of. So the key to a healthy heart is to have the correct balance between LDL and HDL to prevent a build-up of cholesterol. The Western diet which is high in saturated fat, increases LDL which is why Westerners have such a high risk of heart attacks. However a daily dose of fish oil may help to dramatically reduce this risk by increasing our levels of protective HDL-cholesterol. It does this by keeping our levels of another fat, triglyceride, in check.

TRIGLYCERIDES

Triglycerides are found in the saturated fat of meat, milk, butter and cheese. When we eat these foods, the triglycerides are stored in the body and released when we require a sudden burst of energy. In the past, triglycerides would supply people with the energy they needed to keep warm and to cope with hard physical labour. However, today we live in a centrally heated environment, we tend to drive or be driven to work where we sit at a desk all day, finally returning home to relax in front of the television. As a result, we do not need triglycerides to keep us warm or to supply us with extra energy. But our bodies continue to release triglycerides into the bloodstream at times of stress and unless we are physically active, they will not be burned up as energy. Studies have shown that those who have high levels of triglycerides in their bloodstream, have lower than normal levels of HDL which, as we have seen, is needed to control our overall level of cholesterol.

Fortunately, fish oil can help to re-balance HDL and LDL, our good and bad cholesterol, by dramatically reducing the level of triglycerides in our blood. This increases the level of protective HDL-cholesterol and thus reduces our overall blood cholesterol. It was the Eskimos who led scientists to this important discovery. Eskimos, like us, have a diet that is high in saturated animal fat and yet they hardly suffer from heart disease. When Eskimos were examined in their natural environment, their blood cholesterol levels were close to those of people in Britain, but their triglyceride levels were just a quarter of the average UK level. This is highly surprising, as those who eat a lot of animal fat are expected to have high levels of triglycerides in their blood. It was later discovered that it was due to their huge intake of fish oil, that the Eskimos' level of triglycerides were kept under control.

Fish oil can also protect us against heart attacks in another way. Narrowed arteries caused by a build up of cholesterol are not wholly responsible for heart attacks. A heart attack occurs when a blood clot forms blocking the artery, so that the heart is suddenly deprived of its blood supply. It is now thought that an increase in the stickiness of the platelets – gum-like bodies in our blood – is responsible for this fatal blood clot. The stickiness of a platelet depends upon the fatty acids that make up its composition. The usual fatty acids present in platelets tend to promote the release of a particular clotting substance that makes the platelets very sticky. However, a diet rich in fish, or supplemented with fish oil, means that the EPA (eicosapentaenoic acid) present in fish oil enters our platelets instead. This important fatty acid has the opposite effect and makes our platelets much less sticky and, therefore, less likely to clot. Taking fish oil will not prevent our blood from clotting entirely as this would mean that we would bleed to death from a minor cut. It simply appears to reduce the probability of blood clots forming within our arteries, while maintaining its normal ability to stop any bleeding.

In summary

It is thought that fish oil can protect us against heart disease by:

* reducing the level of triglycerides in the blood, thereby increasing the number of HDLs that control the overall cholesterol level.
* reducing the stickiness of blood platelets so that they are less likely to form clots in the arteries.

There have been two highly significant trials into fish oils and heart disease carried out in Britain and America. The Multiple Risk Factor Intervention Trial was conducted between 1973 and 1982 at the Bowman Gray School of Medicine, North Carolina. It involved 12,866 men aged thirty-five to fifty-seven. All the men were at risk from heart disease because of high cholesterol, high blood pressure, or because they were smokers. The men were divided into groups which had to make a variety of different lifestyle changes. One of the groups had to add fish oils to their diet. At the end of the trial, researchers found that the men who had added modest amounts of oily fish to their diet had reduced their risk by 40 percent.

The British study was even more convincing. It was carried out by the Medical Research Council in South Wales and involved 2,000 men who had already had one heart attack and were receiving treatment. The men's treatment differed only in the dietary advice they were given. Some were advised to eat a diet that was low in fat, others were told to increase their fibre intake, especially cereal fibre, and a third group were asked to eat two or three portions of oil-rich fish such as herring or mackerel every week. Those who didn't like fish were asked to take three fish oil capsules a day.

For two years the men were monitored, dietitians even visiting their homes to offer advice and make sure they were sticking to their regime. At the end of the period, nearly 13 percent of the low fat and high fibre groups had died, but, in the fish group the death toll was only 9 percent. These men had already suffered heart damage, yet eating oily fish or taking fish oil supplements for just two years had reduced their death rate by at least 30 percent.

During the 1980s hundreds of medical studies were carried out into the benefits of fish and fish oils. As a result, their role in preventing heart disease is now established as fact.

What Cod Liver Oil Can Do

The research to date shows that fish oils benefit the body in a number of ways. They reduce itchiness and inflammation in skin diseases, ease joint pain, lower blood pressure, and reduce blood fat levels, which in turn reduces the risk of thromboses and heart disease.

Several epidemiological studies have shown that people who eat a lot of fish live longer than those who do not. Japanese people who eat a traditional high-fish diet live longer than the rest of us.

For four consecutive years the Japanese have come top of the international league for long life. That's amazing when you think that most Japanese people live in polluted cities and large towns, are heavy smokers, love salt, lead high stress lifestyles and yet have one-eighth the British rate of heart disease. The same research also revealed that within any one country, people who eat fish live longer than those who do not.

But cod liver and other fish oils don't just mean long life and a healthy heart. Ongoing research continues to show how cod liver oil can benefit the body in many other ways (see Chapter 5). Much of the research into EFAs doesn't concentrate on cod liver oil alone. Some of the studies use mixed fish oils, others use whole oily fish, but both of these combinations contain the same EFAs as cod liver oil. The only significant difference is in concentration.

All this research might lead you to believe that you need to be ill to take cod liver supplements. But its greatest strength lies in its preventative abilities. Taking cod liver oil as a daily supplement could be your simplest insurance plan against ever needing to take it as a remedy. It will help you maintain a healthy heart and circulation and build up your immune system. You'll look great, too – glowing skin, strong nails and shining hair are just some of the beauty perks of taking a daily dose of cod liver oil.

Taking Cod Liver Oil

Potencies vary between capsules, bottled oil and high dose MaxEPA capsules. MaxEPA were produced after research revealed cod liver oil's anti-thrombotic benefits. They are only available on prescription. But, if you can face it, the next best thing is to take the traditional oil. Mixed with either milk or orange juice it doesn't taste bad at all. Oil taken straight has a higher omega-3 content than capsules (0.18g per 1ml as opposed to 0.05g per capsule). Alternatively, you could try one of the orange or lemon flavoured varieties of bottled oil that are now widely available.

The suggested intake of omega-3 long-chain polyunsaturates is one gram a day. You can make this up either in capsules or liquid. If you're choosing capsules look for those that say 'pure fish oil' on the packaging as this means that the oil has not been chemically processed and the basic construction of the omega-3 has been preserved.

YOUR DOSAGE GUIDE

* **Adults and children over one year** – most experts recommend a maximum dose of 10ml (2tsp) although some think you should take as much as 20ml (1tbsp).
* **Arthritis or psoriasis** – you may also need to take 10ml a day.
* **To reduce the risk of a second heart attack** – take at least 3ml of oil daily.
* **Pregnant and breastfeeding women** – take 10–15ml (2–3tsp) a day.
* **Babies 0–6 mths** – ½tsp a day.
* **Babies 7–12 mths** – 1tsp a day.

3

The Link with Arthritis

One of the most heavily researched aspects of cod liver oil is its effect on arthritis. Arthritis is the greatest single cause of disability in Britain. It affects over twenty million people, and anything that can ease the pain and inflammation and improve mobility is welcomed by sufferers of both rheumatoid and osteoarthritis, the two main types of the disease.

Osteoarthritis (OA) is a form of joint disease which affects about five million people in Britain. It tends to start after the age of fifty and affects mostly women. No one really knows what causes it, but it can be brought on by injury, and some forms of the disease seem to have hereditary factors.

Osteoarthritis sets in when the surface of a joint is damaged and the underlying bone reacts abnormally. Knees, hands, hips, big toes, the neck and lower back are the most commonly affected joints. A healthy person's bones are covered at the ends by a thin layer of gristle called cartilage, which allows the joint to move smoothly and acts as a shock absorber so that sudden or jarring movements don't cause pain. Both the cartilage and the end of the bone are further protected by a membrane called the synovial membrane which secretes synovial fluid to lubricate the surfaces and feed the joint. Outside the synovial membrane is a protective capsule and ligaments which keep the joint in place.

When you develop osteoarthritis the cartilage becomes thin and rough and the bone underneath grows thicker and 'bulges', restricting movement in the joint. The synovial membrane tends to become inflamed and produces extra fluid, making the joint swell and become painful. The capsule and ligaments may also thicken and stretch. In severe cases the cartilage can become damaged, exposing the bone underneath, and chalky deposits can form and float around in the fluid. In some cases the joints may become deformed.

Rheumatoid arthritis (RA) is different in that it is an inflammatory condition. The synovial membrane becomes inflamed and there is more swelling and inflammation than there is in osteoarthritis. Inflammation is usually the body's response to injury and helps to get rid of whatever is causing the pain, but in rheumatoid arthritis the inflammation occurs for no reason and appears to be a case of the body's immune system attacking itself. RA also has more widespread effects on the body. It can cause weight loss, anaemia and fatigue, for example. It can strike anyone at any age, but most commonly affects young or middle-aged women.

The first symptoms can occur in the fingers, wrist, or the balls of the feet. The joints swell and become uncomfortable and you can become depressed, irritable and generally unwell. The inflammation may come and go, but eventually it will take its toll on the joint. Constant inflammation can also put pressure on the nerves, causing a tingling or numbing sensation. In severe cases joints can become seriously damaged and unstable. No two people with rheumatoid arthritis are affected in the same way.

Arthritis is usually controlled by non-steroidal anti-inflammatory drugs (NSAIDs), which can cause nausea, indigestion and altered bowel habits, and very occasionally cause bleeding in the stomach. NSAIDs don't actually cure the disease or stop it from spreading; they just reduce pain and inflammation. Diet and physiotherapy also play a part in the treatment and, as a last resort, surgery.

The Codfather

Having arthritis can mean a lifetime of taking prescription drugs just to keep it under control. But many people around the world have found that cod liver oil has greatly improved their chances of leading a full, active and pain-free life. Consequently, most people in Britain who take cod liver oil do so to prevent and treat the pain and stiffness associated with this disease.

Undoubtedly, much of cod liver oil's popularity as an arthritis treatment is due to the work of Dale Alexander, affectionately known as the Codfather. Dale Alexander is an American who worked as a hospital laboratory technician while studying medicine during the war. In 1951 he wrote the first of five books: *Arthritis and Common Sense*. The book told how his romance with cod liver oil was inspired by his mother's ill-health. She was crippled with arthritis and so disillusioned with anything the medical profession had to offer that her son thought he would look for a remedy himself.

By chance he picked up a book that recommended cod liver oil as a cure for rickets. He thought that if it worked for rickets, it would probably work for other diseases of the bone, and began to delve into the folklore of cod liver oil. For maximum effect and minimum taste, he advised taking a tablespoon of cod liver oil mixed with milk or fresh orange juice on an empty stomach. He said the milk or juice cocktail would disguise its three flavours of 'ucky, yucky and bloody awful'.

Alexander's mother took daily doses of cod liver oil and milk, and after six months she reported almost miraculous relief. As a bonus, her hair and skin also improved beyond recognition. Her friends were inspired to try the cod liver oil cocktail and they reported similar success. Alexander has been singing the praises of cod liver oil ever since. Some of his theories may have more in common with nineteenth- rather than twentieth-century science. For example:

Our bodies need lubrication to run smoothly.
Even as a piece of machinery, it needs oil not to get
dried out and rusty.

Nevertheless, he is revered by arthritis sufferers everywhere as the man who brought cod liver oil to the people.

Clinical Evidence

Alexander's beliefs were confirmed by the publication of the first scientific paper on cod liver oil and arthritis, which appeared in a 1959 edition of *The Journal of the National Medicine Association.*

It described a study involving ninety-eight patients who were given a daily dose of 20ml (1tbsp) of cod liver oil mixed with milk or orange juice, taken on an empty stomach. Researchers recorded a 92 percent success rate in relieving pain and swelling and many patients noticed that the condition of their hair, skin and nails also improved.

The researchers involved believed that part of the success of the trial was due to the oil being taken on an empty stomach. This, the dosage and the method were also what Alexander recommended.

Since that first significant trial there have been many others. Several studies have shown that rheumatoid arthritis sufferers receiving a daily intake of long-chain omega-3 polyunsaturates experienced less pain and discomfort. The most recent British study, carried out in 1993, showed that patients with rheumatoid arthritis who took fish oils needed fewer painkillers.

A 1994 double-blind Belgian study involved ninety patients with active rheumatoid arthritis in a twelve-month investigation. The patients were divided into two groups, one taking the equivalent of 10ml cod liver oil a day, the other taking olive oil.

The results showed that those taking the fish oil improved significantly, and their doctors confirmed the improvement. The patients also needed to take fewer drugs to control their condition.

This is significant because many trials are hampered by the painful nature of arthritis. Most patients are on prescription drugs to control pain and inflammation. Understandably, few people suffering chronic pain from a debilitating disease are prepared to stop or reduce their medication to take part in a long-term clinical trial.

However, in an overview of existing studies by JM Kremmer and DR Robinson there was evidence that a regular intake of fish oils brings about significant improvement in swollen joints, levels of fatigue and grip strength. The same review claimed that there was still a need to define the overall therapeutic value of fish oil. It also stated that more evidence was needed on whether patients taking fish oils could come off NSAIDs and slow-acting anti-rheumatic drugs (SAARDs) without any ill-effects. It was stated that, at present, doctors are reluctant to recommend fish oils because of confusion about:

* the amount to prescribe
* the overall effectiveness
* the additional expense of an 'unproven' remedy.

If a study could convince doctors of the undisputed benefits of this unproven remedy then cod liver and other fish oils would be recommended by doctors in the treatment of arthritis. Since recent British research shows that 80 percent of patients at two dietetic clinics in the Midlands would eat more oil-rich fish (and presumably fish oil supplements) if advised to do so by a professional this would surely be regarded as A Good Thing.

So, despite the wealth of clinical trials and testimonials from arthritis sufferers all over the world, cod liver oil is still classified as a food supplement, not a medicine. It has a product licence stating that it can relieve pain and stiffness in joints, but producers can't claim that it cures or helps to treat arthritis. Arthritis sufferers who take the supplement might disagree. There is plenty of both clinical and anecdotal evidence to suggest that it does work. The question is, how?

How Cod Liver Oil Can Help

Cod liver oil has been proved to help damaged and inflamed joints on several levels. Diets that are low in saturated fats or high in essential fatty acids have been shown to benefit arthritis. This is because the body uses essential fatty acids to make chemicals (prostaglandins) which are less inflammatory than those made from the usual dietary fats (leukotrienes). By supplying the body with the raw materials for maintaining less aggressive inflammatory activity cod liver oil can reduce the discomfort of arthritis.

It also contains vitamin D. Lack of vitamin D can cause aches and pains similar to arthritic pains. Cod liver oil on its own cannot undo the damage of arthritis but, combined with gentle exercise and a diet modified to be high in polyunsaturates and low in saturated fats, it can have very positive results.

DIET AND SELF-HELP

* Eat a low-fat diet, high in wholegrains, fibre and heaps of fruit and vegetables. Reduce your salt and alcohol intake as these can cause high blood pressure. Also reduce the amount of red meat, full fat milk and refined sugars in your diet.

* Calcium is important for healthy bones, especially for people with rheumatoid arthritis who are taking high

doses of steroids. Skimmed milk, yoghurt and dark green vegetables should provide adequate calcium. If necessary you can take calcium supplements.

* Selenium is also important. It is an antioxidant that works well with vitamin E to protect the body from disease. It also boosts the immune system.

* Try to keep your weight down, especially if you have arthritis in your hips or legs.

* Regular gentle exercise such as walking, swimming and dancing helps to strengthen the joints and muscles, protecting them from further degeneration.

* Take your daily measure of cod liver oil, either in traditional liquid form mixed with orange juice or milk, or as capsules.

CASE HISTORIES

The famous cookery writer Marguerite Patten began to get stiffness in one knee in 1991 when she was seventy-six years old. In 1992 she also began to get pain in her hip.

*M*y hip was very bad indeed and my knee was terribly swollen. I had extreme pain, and my movement was restricted a great deal. I had awful nights when my leg was just locked, so that I would have needed a crane to come down from the ceiling to lift me out of bed. My doctor told me it was arthritis and I would need an X-ray to determine what treatment would be necessary.

I went to the Nuffield hospital for an X-ray and they immediately told me I needed a hip replacement. They said both my hip and knee were very bad. I thought they were making a fuss about nothing, but my doctor agreed that I had to have a hip replacement.

I would never contemplate a hip replacement and I don't like to take pills. I told them I hadn't time to have an operation. My husband wasn't well and I'm desperately busy. In any case I decided arthritis was not going to ruin my life and I'd have a good old fight.

I have great faith in acupuncture, but in this case it was a great disappointment. It did not help as much as I had hoped it would and it took a long time to get there and back. I'm too busy to spend a whole morning once a week on acupuncture, especially if it's not that beneficial.

I was still in a lot of pain, so I bought all the diet books I could find and they all contradicted each other. An American one said to eat liver often, others said eat no meat at all. I followed them to a degree. I stopped drinking alcohol, soft drinks, tea and coffee for about a month and I started taking one capsule of cod liver oil every day.

I'd read about the benefits of cod liver oil and as I was willing to try anything, I gave it a go. That month really turned the scales.

I have been taking cod liver oil capsules now for about a year and a half and I am a very different person. I still have arthritis, but it doesn't interfere with anything I want to do. I do have some pain at night but there is a vast difference between that and lying there in agony not knowing how you are going to move your leg. I never have nights like that any more. If I sit for hours and hours, stand cooking for a very long time or don't take any exercise I get a bit stiff, but it goes when I get up and move around. The only problem I have is going upstairs. Going down the stairs and walking are fine. I'm an ardent gardener, and I can manage without any bother.

I have painkilling and anti-inflammatory tablets, but I have only had nine in nine months. There are days when I have absolutely no pain at all. I'm seventy-nine and I work a full week. I've written 162 books. I write for four magazines, do a page in a paper every week and I'm doing television. I behave as I have done all my working life. I couldn't have done all this if I felt as I did in 1992.

Sam Slipman, an eighty-year old shopkeeper who lives in Hertfordshire, has beaten arthritis with a combination of cod liver oil and exercise.

i've got osteoarthritis, which is caused by wear and tear mostly – spondylitis of the spine, to be exact. I was in my forties when I got it. I was admitted to the Orthopaedic Hospital at Stanmore and had manipulation which aggravated it so that I couldn't move my neck or head at all. I was put on traction for a couple of weeks and I had to have cortisone injections in my spine every week. They were so painful I had to have them under anaesthetic.

It was very bad at that time, but I have alleviated most of the pain by exercising and taking cod liver oil. I take cod liver oil because it helps to reduce inflammation and builds up my energy levels. I take two teaspoons of it in soya milk every morning. It's something I read about in a book by Dale Alexander some years ago. I find that the traditional liquid acts much more quickly than the capsules.

I exercise religiously every day and that keeps me active. I occasionally take painkillers, but I got rid of the several types of painkillers I used to take years ago because they upset my stomach. I feel well now, the combination of exercise and cod liver oil definitely helps.

I produce leaflets and have made a video to help other sufferers and I get great pleasure from hearing from people who have benefited from my regime. In fact I read in the paper recently that the Queen had arthritis in her hand from so much handshaking. I sent her a copy of my video and leaflets and received a very nice letter back thanking me, but saying I shouldn't believe everything I read in the newspapers.

4

Common Skin Disorders

Cod liver oil has been used to treat skin diseases for at least 100 years. In 1877 Tilbury Fox, an eminent London dermatologist, wrote in his *Atlas of Skin Diseases*, 'if eczema be present, cod liver oil should be given freely,' and for prurigo – a severe type of itching – he said, 'no remedy is as good as cod liver oil'.

Up until the 1930s or 1940s, many dermatologists would have agreed with Fox that cod liver and other dietary oils were the best treatment for eczema and other skin diseases. But the drug industry was growing fast and the arrival of steroid creams around this time put paid to cod liver oil treatment. Twenty years later, steroids also seemed to have run their course, for in the 1970s the side-effects of steroid use became widely known and many people refused to use them; even doctors were afraid to prescribe them. Science then turned back to nature for a helping hand in controlling uncomfortable, embarrassing and often disfiguring skin conditions.

The Role of Skin

As the largest organ in the body our skin has an important role to play. It holds all our internal organs neatly in place, helps to keep the body at a steady temperature, acts as an efficient elimination system and also as a sensor to changes in our environment. But even though it protects us, its sensitivity makes it vulnerable.

Skin is an accurate barometer of the state of our health – it is often the first part of the body to react to both external and internal changes. Its colour and texture are a good indication of its condition. Smooth, supple, glowing skin is the ideal, but our genetic inheritance plus abuse from stress, illness, diet, hormones, the environment and cosmetics make it difficult to achieve and maintain that ideal. Spots, blotches and rashes are minor imperfections which most of us expect from time to time, but chronic conditions such as eczema and psoriasis are much more distressing and difficult to deal with.

Psoriasis

Psoriasis is an inflammatory disease that affects about 2 percent of people in Britain. It was made famous by Dennis Potter's *Singing Detective*. Anyone who saw the television programme will have some idea of what torture severe psoriasis can be. Not everyone is so badly affected, but even those who have a mild form of the condition experience pain, discomfort and often severe embarrassment about their appearance. Unfortunately, as with most skin conditions, anxiety can make it worse.

Psoriasis appears as thickened red patches of inflamed skin, often covered in silvery scales, that can bleed when scratched. Psoriasis can cause discomfort and itching as it spreads over the body – knees, elbows, scalp, trunk and back are common sites – and sometimes sufferers also have painful, inflamed joints. The condition tends to appear between the ages of ten and thirty, when it is likely to be most embarrassing. Nobody knows exactly why some people get psoriasis although there are several theories. It does seem to involve hereditary factors, and it is known that it can occur due to the overactivity of various body functions. One of these abnormalities is in the way the body processes essential fatty acids, another is in the reaction to free-radicals.

The inflamed patches of skin which characterise psoriasis occur because of an abnormality of skin cell production. New cells are produced about ten times faster than normal, but the old cells are shed at the normal rate. As a result live cells clump into thickened patches of inflammation covered with dead flaking skin. Such attacks can be triggered by stress, illness and damage to the skin. Conventional medical treatment involves using ultra-violet light, emollient creams and, in cases where it is accompanied by arthritis, NSAIDs. More severe cases are sometimes treated by powerful drugs made from derivatives of vitamin A. These treatments can help to alleviate the symptoms but they don't tackle the root of the problem. People with psoriasis are expected to resign themselves to the fact that there is no cure.

HOW COD LIVER OIL CAN HELP

Cod liver oil reduces both the severity and the extent of the effects of psoriasis. It does this in two ways: by its vitamin content and, more importantly, because of its high levels of EFAs. In summary:

* **Vitamin A** has been proved to combat psoriasis because it inhibits the formation of polamines (toxic amino acids) which are what make the skin cells reproduce so quickly.

* **Vitamin E** improves the texture of the skin and speeds the healing process, helping to regulate the rate at which cells reproduce. It is also a powerful antioxidant, so it helps prevent internal skin cell damage and can delay premature skin ageing.

* **EPA** can help to reduce inflammation. It does this by providing the material which the body needs to make prostaglandins, which are essential for healthy tissues.

Prostaglandins can also be made from another fatty acid called arachidonic acid (AA), but this is more likely to cause inflammation than EPA. AA has long been implicated in the inflammation associated with psoriasis. If the body is supplied with sufficient EPA it can make prostaglandins which reduce the inflammatory effects of those made from AA.

✱ **Fish oil** may counteract one side-effect of the retinoic acid (vitamin A)-derived drugs which are sometimes used to treat severe psoriasis. These drugs can cause serum triglyceride levels to rise. In many ways triglycerides are similar to cholesterol and high levels can increase the risk of heart disease.

✱ **Omega-3s** also improve blood flow by slightly thinning the blood and improving the elasticity of red blood cells. Free-flowing blood carries more oxygen to nourish the skin.

THE EVIDENCE

Research began in Greenland, where Eskimos were found to have a much lower rate of psoriasis than Europeans. Since then clinical trials have proved the benefit of fish oils in controlling the spread, appearance and intensity of the disease. In one study, psoriasis patients benefited from taking fish oil supplements for eight weeks. In a more recent trial eight out of ten patients with psoriasis improved after taking EPA supplements for six weeks.

In a significant 1988 British study at The Royal Hallamshire Hospital in Sheffield, twenty-eight patients with chronic psoriasis completed a twelve-week double-blind clinical trial. The patients had to continue with their usual prescribed topical treatment and stick to their normal diet. They were divided into two groups: one group was asked to take ten MaxEPA cod liver oil capsules a day; the other, ten capsules of olive oil. Both sets of capsules looked the same and their taste was disguised by peppermint. The study lasted for twelve weeks and patients were assessed at four-weekly intervals for improvements in the effects of the disease.

* **Itching:** at eight and twelve weeks the MaxEPA group had significantly less itching, but there was no change in the olive oil control group.

* **Red patches:** again, at eight and twelve weeks the MaxEPA group showed significant improvement, while there was no change in the control group.

* **Scaling:** by eight weeks the scaling had improved in the MaxEPA group, but that improvement was not significantly better than in the control group.

* **Surface area:** there was a trend towards improvement in the MaxEPA group, but there was no significant improvement in the control group.

In 1993 a German ten-day study involving twenty male and female patients who were hospitalised with acute psoriasis demonstrated the greater benefits to be had from fish oil. They were divided into two groups: one received intravenous treatment with omega-3 EFAs (derived from fish oil); the other received the same treatment with omega-6 EFAs (derived from soya oil). Within ten days the symptoms of patients on omega-3 treatment had improved by 45–76 percent, while the omega-6 group had improved by 16–25 percent.

The researchers concluded that, in addition to the benefits of taking fish oils regularly for chronic psoriasis, concentrated

EPA or DHA may turn out to be a new therapeutic way to alleviate the symptoms of acute psoriasis and other inflammatory skin diseases.

Research has shown that, at the very least, taking fish oil supplements along with drug treatment can bring about an immediate improvement in psoriasis. Also, the side-effects of anti-cancer drugs, which are sometimes used to treat the more severe cases of psoriasis, can be blocked by taking EFAs.

CASE HISTORY

Elaine Barnett, from Wakering, Essex, is fifty-three and has had psoriasis for thirty years. She has been taking two fish oil capsules every day for the last three years.

*P*soriasis has a very strong emotional link. I had it first when I was twenty-three. I was pregnant at the time and my brother had just been killed in a car accident. I think the emotional impact of both events together had a lot to do with bringing it to the surface.

I had very large patches about four or five inches wide on my legs and feet and I also had it on my ears, on my scalp, on my pelvis, elbows and knees – everywhere really!

My doctor gave me cortisone creams but I didn't want to use them. I used to scratch the patches sometimes until they bled and I didn't like the idea of cortisone going into my blood stream. After that I just gave up on medical treatment and tried to live with it.

The fish oil cure came about by accident. I started taking it to try to bring down my then high cholesterol level. I've got this ambition to live to 100 you see, so I always take vitamins and supplements.

As a happy side-effect of taking fish oil the patches of psoriasis started to go, one by one. This was a very gradual process and now I've just got small patches on my knees and elbows. Over the last year several people have said, 'Elaine, you don't have psoriasis any more!' Of course, I still do, but that's how much it has diminished.

Fish oil is the only thing that has had any effect on my psoriasis. It has improved the quality of my skin generally, it's much less dry and obviously, as I get older, that's a real plus.

Eczema

Eczema is a general term for chronic skin conditions characterised by inflamed, itchy, red scaly patches and blisters. There are two main types: atopic eczema and contact dermatitis.

ATOPIC ECZEMA
Common in babies on the face, creases of the elbows, neck, knees and bottom. Most children grow out of the condition by their teens, but that's of little comfort to a child who is in agony with itchy, cracked and bleeding skin. This type of eczema can occur for no known reason, but it can also run in families, especially where there is an inherited tendency towards asthma or hay fever. Conventional treatment ranges from simple emollients to prevent the skin from cracking to steroid, antibiotic and antihistamine drugs. Stress, anxiety and some foods such as chocolates, oranges, nuts and milk are believed to make symptoms worse. Unfortunately, like psoriasis, there is no cure.

ECZEMA AND DIET
Many skin specialists believe that diet has an important part to play in controlling eczema. Certain foods cause intolerance or allergies which can exacerbate existing skin disorders such as eczema. The foods that are often to blame are dairy produce – milk, butter, cheese, etc. or wheat, nuts, tomatoes and fish.

Essential Fatty Acid Metabolism

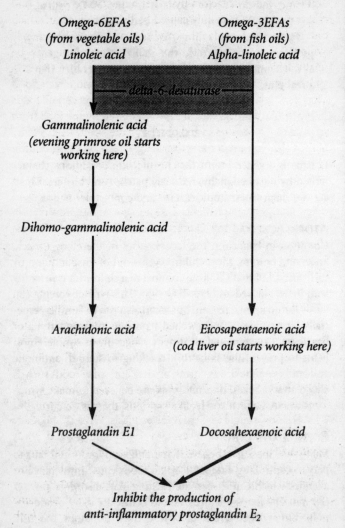

Omega-6EFAs
(from vegetable oils)
Linoleic acid

Omega-3EFAs
(from fish oils)
Alpha-linoleic acid

— delta-6-desaturase —

Gammalinolenic acid
(evening primrose oil starts
working here)

Dihomo-gammalinolenic acid

Arachidonic acid

Eicosapentaenoic acid
(cod liver oil starts working here)

Prostaglandin E1

Docosahexaenoic acid

Inhibit the production of
anti-inflammatory prostaglandin E$_2$

However, it must be stressed that eczema may be provoked by other very different factors than diet alone. Some people find that their eczema is mainly caused by dairy produce, in which case it is easy to improve the condition of their skin by simply avoiding milk, cheese, etc. For others, the cause may be unavoidable environmental factors such as house dust mites, in which case, giving up dairy produce will have no effect. Food allergies are very individual, but if you suspect that certain foods may provoke your eczema, it is worth excluding the food from your diet for a week or so and observing the effect. Keep a diary of the foods you eat, writing down any effects on the condition of your skin. Bear in mind that if you stop eating dairy produce or other important foods, you will be depriving your body of calcium and other nutrients which you will need to get from other foods or supplements instead. For more information about eczema read my *Quick Guide to Dry Skin and Eczema* (Boxtree, £3.99).

CONTACT DERMATITIS
Usually an allergic reaction to something your skin comes into contact with – maybe washing-up liquid, a metal watch strap or the mouse on your computer. Again treatment is usually with a low-dose steroid cream and you are advised to avoid the irritating substance or material as much as possible.

HOW COD LIVER OIL CAN HELP
There is not as much clinical evidence for the benefits of cod liver oil in treating eczema as there is for psoriasis. What studies there are tend to conflict. However, a 1987 double-blind study reported in the *British Journal of Dermatology* proved that supplementing with MaxEPA capsules did have some clinical benefit.

Sixteen people with eczema were given 10g of MaxEPA every day for twelve weeks, while a control group spent the same period of time on a placebo. At the end of the period both groups were assessed for severity of symptoms. When the patients assessed their own condition, those on fish oil claimed significant improvement compared to the placebo group. However, the assessors found only marginal differences between the two groups. Nevertheless, some improvement was shown to have occurred.

Unfortunately, most trials involving essential fatty acids and eczema have concentrated on oils from the omega-6 family, in particular evening primrose oil, so it is difficult to prove a case for cod liver oil on the basis of clinical evidence alone. The most encouraging information is anecdotal, coming from people with eczema who find that cod liver oil either alone or in conjunction with other supplements makes a real improvement to their skin.

One theory about eczema is that people who have it experience a blockage in the first stage of the process that converts essential fatty acids into a form that can be used by the body. All processes within the body are controlled by the activity of enzymes. It is the job of specific enzymes to convert the alpha-linoleic acid in vegetable oil, and the linolenic acid in fish oil, into other substances that the body can use. In the case of cod liver oil, the enzyme delta-6-desaturase converts alpha-linolenic acid into eicosapentaenoic acid which eventually ends up as docosahexaenoic acid. The linoleic acid in vegetable oil is also converted using the delta-6-desaturase enzyme into gamma linolenic acid and this in turn becomes arachidonic acid. It has been discovered that the activity of this important enzyme is inhibited in eczema sufferers who are, therefore, unable to create GLA and EPA themselves.

However, supplementing their diet with fish oil and evening primrose oil can overcome this problem as these oils contain eicosapentaenoic acid and gamma-linolenic acid respectively. Therefore, the body does not need to convert linolenic and linoleic acid from other food sources into the more important

DHA and GLA. Both of these EFAs are thought to improve the condition of eczema because GLA is converted by enzymes into prostaglandin E1 which inhibits the production of prostaglandin E2. Likewise, the DHA in cod liver oil inhibits the production of this inflammatory prostaglandin. In this respect, cod liver oil and evening primrose oil work well together and it is possible to buy supplements that contain a mixture of both.

The current thinking in both eczema and psoriasis is that fish oils are most effective when combined with other forms of treatment, but this is an area that still has to be researched. Both omega-6s and omega-3s seem capable of improving eczema independently, but more often than not they work more effectively when used together. If one used the diet of Eskimos as the recipe for perfect skin, then a combination of cod liver oil and evening primrose oil comes closer to mimicking their EFA levels than fish oils alone.

CASE HISTORY

Thirty-two-year-old Pat Hamilton developed eczema ten years ago just after she had completed her university degree course. Around the same time she moved to London from a small seaside town in Wales.

i'd always had good skin, so I was distressed when I started to get itchy red patches of eczema on my scalp and eyebrows, around my hairline and under my eyes. It looked and felt dreadful. My doctor prescribed a mild hydrocortisone cream which cleared up the angry outbreaks, but I didn't like to use it too often on my face as it thins the skin.

One day in my local library I picked up a copy of Dale Alexander's *Dry Skin and Common Sense* and that got me started on the cod liver oil cocktail. Every morning I would mix a tablespoon of cod liver oil with orange juice, hold my nose and down it in one. My flat mate thought I'd lost my sense of taste but if you hold your nose you can't taste the oil.

I did this every morning for about two years and then reduced it to two teaspoons every other day. The improvement was very gradual. I can't pin-point a time when my skin improved, but I hardly ever have an eczema attack now. In fact, I've still got the tube of hydrocortisone cream I was prescribed in 1986!

Funnily enough I also get hay fever, not because of pollen, I think it's got to do with traffic pollution in the summer. I started getting it after I had glandular fever about six years ago. But this last couple of summers it hasn't bothered me. I don't know if I've outgrown it or if the cod liver oil has put paid to that, too.

My eczema hasn't vanished, it sometimes reappears at times of extreme stress or when I'm particularly low, but on a day-to-day basis, it's not a problem.

Acne, Spots and Dry Skin Conditions

Acne, spots, blackheads, whiteheads and dry skin conditions may not be the inevitable consequence of teenage hormones in turmoil; they are just as likely to be caused by a lack of vitamins A and E, zinc and EFAs. If your diet is high in saturated fats such as those found in red meat, and chemically altered unsaturated fats such as those in some margarines, your skin will probably suffer from clogged and infected pores. Healthy skin depends on fats that 'flow'. Free-flowing fish and evening primrose oils make up the complete family of EFAs that are needed for fabulous skin.

The vitamin A and E content in cod liver oil also makes it perfect for keeping skin looking and feeling its best. Vitamin A helps to prevent and/or correct dry, rough and scaly skin and scalp. Lack of vitamin A can kill off new cells before they reach the surface. This can also lead to blocked pores, blackheads, spots and acne.

Most brands of cod liver oil are enriched with the antioxidant vitamin E. In the body vitamin E protects both vitamin A and the polyunsaturated fats needed to keep skin moist. It also defends healthy tissues from the damaging effects of free-radicals. Free-radicals can cause premature ageing of the skin by damaging the collagen and elastin fibres that keep it plump and taut. They can also interfere with skin cell reproduction, leading to a dull, blotchy complexion.

There have been surprisingly few studies into the role of EFAs in preventing or clearing acne, but the low levels of EFAs found in the sebum of people with acne seem to indicate that EFA deficiency may be the cause of the blocked follicles and covering of dead skin cells that trigger the spots. This is similar to the theory of how EFA deficiency causes the red scaly patches in eczema.

As early as 1958, an experimental study reported in the *British Medical Bulletin* showed that EFA deficiency was responsible for the skin losing water, which is a feature of acne. Probably more importantly it claimed that lack of EFAs may also cause the characteristic layers of dead and hardened skin that cover blocked follicles in cases of acne. Removing this dead and hardened skin is an important part of acne treatment. Many modern acne drugs are designed to do just that, as this simultaneously clears the blocked follicles that cause acne spots.

If cod liver oil can do from the inside what potentially damaging drug treatment can do from the outside, we might all look forward to better skin.

——— 5 ———
Future Benefits

As research reveals an increasingly impressive list of benefits from improved nutrition and EFAs in particular, the once magical properties of cod liver oil are gaining scientific acceptance in many different areas of medicine.

Clinical trials into the effects of cod liver oil on heart disease and inflammatory diseases of the skin and joints continue to come up with convincing evidence that cod liver oil can make a real contribution to preventing and controlling these diseases. Ever more amazing claims are being made outside clinical research. Enthusiasts report remarkable positive side-effects such as healthier, shinier, thicker and faster-growing hair, glowing skin, stronger nails, even less sunburn. Other claims, such as the reports of increased sex drive remain as eyebrow-raising anecdotes. However, the anecdotes of today may well be the clinical findings of tomorrow!

Research is widening into areas which have not previously been associated with cod liver oil. Fish oils generally may prove useful in counteracting the side-effects of certain drugs such as cyclosporins, which are used after organ transplants so that the recipient's immune system doesn't reject the donated organ. Oils have also been shown to reduce high blood pressure and may ultimately prove to be a better long-term treatment than the continued use of beta-blockers. In laboratory studies, cod liver oil has also been shown to help burns to heal, just as older generations used it to heal scars. In clinical trials it has also helped to ease the symptoms of ulcerative colitis and reduce sufferers' need for steroids.

And, of course, just as those old wives' tales claimed, fish is good for our brains because of its DHA content. Dr Michael Crawford of the Institute of Brain Chemistry and Human Nutrition has explained why essential fatty acids are so essential:

> *Fish and seafoods have played a singularly important part throughout the ages. Indeed new evidence points to the high probability that they were an essential component to the evolution of the human brain and therefore vital to our present health and the health of our children.*

It seems likely that in the future a whole range of diseases will be prevented and treated with this ancient natural cure. Some areas are already being explored as likely to benefit from the unique properties of the omega-3 oils found in cod liver oil.

Bonny Babies

We know from the example of war babies that cod liver oil can help children grow up stronger and healthier. But in the 1950s no one really understood why. Since then, observations of babies born to women in the Faroe Islands have shown that fish eaters tend to have bigger babies than the international average. The researchers Olsen and Joensen could find no explanation at the time, but since then it has been attributed to the high levels of omega-3s in the diet.

In 1993 researchers from the London School of Hygiene and Tropical Medicine took a closer look at the diet of pregnant women in the Faroe Islands. They looked at how often 1,000 women ate fish during their pregnancy and compared the information with the average weight and length of newborns. Factors such as age, weight, height, marital status and smoking habits were all taken into account. The result showed that women who ate three seafish meals a week had slightly longer pregnancies and bigger, heavier babies than those who didn't eat fish.

Babies also need EFAs. It has become accepted that the essential fatty acids DHA and AA are important for a child's early development. DHA, for example, is vital for the health of the brain, eyes and nervous system. Newborn babies don't have a fully developed nervous system at birth. EFAs are transferred to the baby in the womb from the placenta and, after birth, are also available in breast milk. Formula feeds do not contain EFAs.

It is estimated that 80 percent of a newborn's DHA levels accumulate during the last three months of pregnancy. For this reason, premature babies are particularly vulnerable to DHA deficiency. If they are then fed infant formula, they quickly lose what levels of DHAs they have. The outcome of all this is that premature babies can have poorer visual and, possibly, cognitive development than their full-term counterparts, and the developmental damage done in the early weeks of life appears to be permanent. Some researchers believe that even full-term babies fed on infant formulae may have lower levels of DHA than those who are breastfed.

This is an area that needs further investigation. Recent German research concluded that, although it is desirable to have an infant formula that is as close as possible to breast milk, the potential for side-effects and the cost of such a venture need to be closely examined. EFAs are susceptible to oxidisation, say researchers Decsi and Koletzko, and adding them to a formula may endanger a baby's levels of protective antioxidants. Even if this problem is overcome, it is felt that the venture may prove too expensive. It is not clear whether vitamins A and E present in cod liver oil adequately make up for the shortfall in the natural level of antioxidants.

Note: When taking cod liver oil it is important that pregnant women do not exceed the recommended dose. Cod liver oil is rich in vitamin A and excessive amounts of this vitamin could cause birth defects.

Asthma and Hay Fever

Asthma is yet another distressing disease that seems to have become more widespread recently. Recurrent attacks of wheezing and breathlessness can range in degree from the barely noticeable to the life-threatening. Again, there is no cure, although sufferers and doctors alike are desperate that one should be found. Hay fever, too, is on the increase as our bodies seem to become more sensitive to pollution from car fumes and seemingly harmless substances such as pollen and dust.

The anti-inflammatory properties of cod liver oil have also been put to the test in treating people with asthma, with mixed results. It started from an investigation into whether EPA and DHA could suppress inflammatory and immune responses by competing with those aggressive inflammatory agents, leukotrienes. Two studies carried out in the mid-1980s concluded that taking fish oil supplements every day may reduce inflammation.

One of those studies was by Professor Tak Lee at Guy's Hospital in London, who investigated the benefits of EPA and DHA in the treatment of allergic asthma. He discovered that asthmatics, unlike the rest of the population, have detectable levels of leukotrienes in their lungs. These cause inflammation and are involved in triggering an asthmatic response when a sufferer comes into contact with pollen or other allergens.

Leukotrienes can be made from either arachidonic acid or EPA and, as with prostaglandins, those made from AA are the more aggressive of the two. Professor Lee observed the effect of fish oil supplements on asthmatics who were exposed to known allergens and recorded that they had far fewer asthma attacks than when they had previously come into contact with these allergens.

Leukotrienes have also been detected in the noses of hay fever sufferers when they are under attack. Future research might show that cod liver oil may also play a part in hay fever control.

Skin and Bone

Eighteenth- and nineteenth-century skeletons unearthed during building work in London may hold the secret to strong bones and firm skin. Researcher Theya Mollesen of the Natural History Museum has concluded that our female ancestors had stronger bones and better collagen structures than we have, probably because they had a high fish and shellfish diet.

More evidence of the bone-strengthening properties of omega-3s comes from Japan. Sakaguchi and colleagues fed a number of laboratory rats on a variety of diets and then measured the weight and strength of their bones. The researchers found that the rats fed on a diet that included fish oils had much heavier, stronger bones than the rest, even when they were low in calcium. The researchers concluded that omega-3s may prove to be the vital link in preventing osteo-porosis.

Osteoporosis is something that many women fear. It causes the skeleton to shrink so that skin sags and, more importantly, it makes you more susceptible to fractures and broken bones.

On average bones start to lose their density after the age of thirty-five, but not significantly, until oestrogen production from the ovaries stops after the menopause. Osteoporosis is so talked about that many women may think of it as an inevitable result of ageing, just like wrinkles or grey hair. This is not true. The way you live and the food you eat can make an enormous difference to whether or not you get osteoporosis. Exercise matters, as does vitamin D and EFA intake.

Regular weight-bearing exercise, such as walking, dancing or swimming is a great bone booster. Vitamin D is important because it helps your body utilise calcium in bone remineralisation through activating the thyroid and parathyroid hormones.

EFAs are needed to make prostaglandins which have a powerful effect on hormone balance. Osteoporosis is specifically related to a drop in hormone levels after the menopause, so fish (omega-3) and vegetable oils (omega-6) are both needed to help the body make the balance of hormones needed to keep you healthy.

Maybe a daily dose of cod liver oil will give us the same bone benefits as our fish-eating ancestors.

... AND TEETH

Two Australian researchers, Littleton and Frohlich, have also been examining old bones, this time from the Arabian Gulf. The jaw bones from these samples, which range from between 500 and 5,000 years old, have been related to the type of food that would have been available to those people at that time.

The researchers found that the jaw bones from the fish-eating communities had better teeth, less decay and fewer missing molars than the jawbones taken from inland farming areas where fish would not have been available.

Multiple Sclerosis

During the last few years there has been some positive research into the benefits of EFAs in the treatment of multiple sclerosis (MS). MS is a disease of the central nervous system which tends to strike young people, between teenage and middle-age, peaking in the early thirties. It is more common in temperate climates, especially among women. It is unknown among Eskimos and native Americans and is uncommon among Chinese and Japanese.

Diagnosing and treating the disease is hampered by the fact that nobody fully understands what it is and how it develops. It also tends to stop and start, especially in the early stages, and this makes it difficult to judge the effect of particular treatments.

But what does seem clear is that it can benefit from EFAs. EFAs are elements in the myelin sheath which is made up of fats and protein and forms the protective covering of nerve fibre. Inflammation of and damage to the myelin sheath are at the core of MS.

Some studies have shown that MS sufferers have low levels of EFAs, which can be corrected within a year by EFA supplements. In the case of MS they seem able to protect against an attack and repair the damage should an attack occur.

Many people with MS say that supplementing with a combination of omega-3 and omega-6 EFAs is beneficial. When you consider that 60 percent of the brain is made up of structural fats, rich in EFAs, and that these form the building blocks of the central nervous system, it's easy to see how important cod liver oil could be. Again, this is an area of ongoing research.

Cod Liver Oil Protects Smokers

Nobody can be left in any doubt that smoking kills. And one of the major causes of death in smokers is chronic obstructive pulmonary disease (COPD). This is the collective term for chronic bronchitis and emphysema. Scientists don't completely understand how smoking causes COPD, but it does seem to have inflammatory characteristics which may be dampened by omega-3 essential fatty acids.

Dr Eyal Shahar and colleagues at the University of Minnesota recently studied the effects of omega-3 in 8,960 smokers and ex-smokers. They found that smokers who ate fish two or three times a week had two-thirds the risk of developing chronic bronchitis and one-third the risk of emphysema compared with those who had fish less than once a week. The researchers concluded that a regular high intake of omega-3s may protect smokers against some common types of lung disease. This should not, however, delay a decision to stop smoking.

Strokes – A Thing of the Past?

Based on the research into the Eskimo diet, it was once believed that the anti-clotting properties of high levels of omega-3 could increase the risk of stroke. But the latest information from the Zutphen study, a long-term follow-up, has contradicted this belief.

In 1970, the researchers obtained cross-check dietary histories from 552 men between the ages of fifty and sixty-nine. They monitored the men for fifteen years and found that those who ate an average of 35g of fish a day had only half the risk of dying of a stroke as those who ate less than 20g a day. The risks did not change even when they made allowances for smoking, drinking alcohol or other known risk factors. The researchers concluded that at least one portion of fish a week can reduce your risk of stroke. On this basis low levels of cod liver oil would confer the same benefits.

Heart Disease and Thrombosis

Coronary heart disease accounts for a significant number of deaths among diabetics. It is accepted that omega-3 can reduce the risk of heart disease among other high-risk groups and studies in Sweden and Denmark show that they could have a similar effect on diabetics. The same research revealed that omega-3s can also reduce the risk of thrombosis. Research into this area is ongoing and controversial.

One of the effects of thrombosis can be an increased heart beat as the heart tries to compensate for the slowing down in circulation. This irregular beating can often prove fatal.

New research from America shows that fish oils have the potential to reduce this rapid beating in hearts undergoing simulated heart attacks. This research confirms the earlier DART study, which showed that there were fewer deaths among men who had already had one heart attack when they ate an oily fish diet, than those who followed other dietary regimes.

A trial is under way currently to investigate whether taking regular levels of fish oils will reduce the risk of a first heart attack in people with angina. Omega-3s are known to be effective against angina, which is accepted as an early sign of heart disease. It is logical to assume that an improvement in the condition of angina sufferers could prevent them from ever having a heart attack. Results of this trial will not be available for some time.

Cancer Cure?

Finding a cure for cancer would undoubtedly be one of the greatest medical breakthroughs of the century. We know already that diet plays an enormous part in whether or not we get cancer. According to the Bristol Cancer Help Centre the type of diet you eat appears as a significant factor in up to 45 percent of all cancers.

If cod liver oil can help to alleviate or lessen the risk of getting so many other diseases, it is possible that it may also help with cancer. Research in this area is still in its infancy, but preliminary work into the effects of cod liver oil on laboratory mice has shown positive results.

At the University of Texas, scientists conducted comparative tests using corn oil and fish oil on cancerous tumours from at least four organs. At the end of the trial the tumours of the mice that had been on the fish oil diet had diminished while the tumours of those on the corn oil had grown. This trial showed that fish oil may prove to be beneficial, particularly in treating breast cancer.

Similar research showed that EPA, specifically, slowed the growth of tumours in laboratory animals and had the added benefit of preventing weight loss. The results suggest that EPA as the pure fatty acid should be considered for clinical trials as both a preventative against weight loss and malnutrition in people with cancer and also as an anti-tumour agent.

There is still a long way to go in this area of research, but further trials are under way in the United States.

These are just a few of the areas where cod liver oil is being researched as a natural medicine. Many people don't need to be convinced of its benefits, but all areas of medicine must be exhaustively researched to ensure that we get the best and safest treatments possible. Cod liver oil has come a long way from seventeenth-century rheumatic rub to natural remedy of the 1990s. Its many benefits are as vital today as they were hundreds of years ago. As an important part of our diet, and perhaps as a future medicine, it could help us all live a long and healthy life.

In Brief

The omega-3 essential fatty acids, abundant in cod liver oil, fight heart disease by reducing:

* blood fat levels
* blood pressure

* blood thickness
* blood clotting.

They also:
* stabilise heart beat
* develop a healthy nervous system, brain function and eyesight in unborn and premature babies, and help combat diseases of the nervous system such as MS
* help to balance an overactive immune system which causes inflammatory diseases such as rheumatoid arthritis, psoriasis, ulcerative colitis and possibly MS and allergies.

6

The Oil Fish Diet

Many of the benefits we get from cod liver oil can also be received from eating other oily fish such as mackerel and herring. Oily fish are the richest source of omega-3 essential fatty acids so we should make them a regular part of our diet. Unfortunately, as a nation we do not eat much fresh fish and this is reflected in our general health. Britain has one of the highest rates of heart disease, and eczema and psoriasis affect a considerable portion of the population as well. In order to discover the reasons behind this scientists have carried out vast epidemiological studies to compare the differences in diet and lifestyle between various countries and the risk of developing certain diseases in those countries.

As a result of these studies, it is known that the Mediterraneans, like the Eskimos, have a far lower rate of heart disease which is thought to be due to a diet rich in essential fatty acids in the form of fish and vegetable oils. Fresh, unrefined fish, fruit and vegetables are abundant in the rural areas of France, Italy, Spain and Greece and many scientists are of the opinion that it is the combination of these natural foods which is responsible for the good health of these nations.

Unfortunately, it is a different story here in Britain, where we tend to favour meat over fish. Meat contains saturated fat which, in large amounts, will increase the depositing of cholesterol in the arteries, raising the risk of heart attacks and thrombosis. Almost one-third of us will die from heart disease and it is Britain's biggest killer of both men and women. However, this appallingly high figure can be reduced by a general move to a healthier diet rich in fresh fish, fruit and vegetables and low in animal fats.

This is not as easy for us as it is for the Mediterraneans, who are surrounded by olive groves, fruit trees and fish freshly caught from their shores. For those who live in urban areas of Britain, the supermarket is the main source of food and we are often tempted to take the easy option when shopping by selecting preserved pre-packed foods and ready-made meals. These may taste good, but they have very little nutritional value due to the processing methods. It is far better for us to create our own meals using fresh ingredients, and fish makes a very simple and versatile dish. The larger supermarkets now offer a variety of fresh fish and it is worth searching for your local fishmonger who will have a much wider selection.

However, not all fish contain the fatty acids which are so good for us. Merely having the odd fishfinger is not going to provide much protection against heart disease or improve the condition of our skin. Oily fish such as sardines and mackerel are needed to boost our levels of EPA and DHA, so that our bodies will be better equipped to protect us against a whole host of degenerative illnesses. Some of the best sources of these omega-3 EFAs are:

* Anchovies
* Bass
* Carp
* Cod
* Haddock
* Halibut
* Herring
* Lake trout
* Mackerel
* Mullet
* Rainbow trout

* Red snapper
* Salmon
* Sardines
* Sole
* Sprats
* Squid
* Swordfish
* Tuna.

Note: Tuna should be bought fresh and not tinned, as the fish oil is drained off and replaced with refined vegetable oils.

Choosing the Right Fish

Many of the wet fish available in supermarkets and fish shops, particularly trout, have been spawned and reared in special hatcheries and farms. These fish are fed soya meals or grain which contains little or none of the omega-3 EFAs that plankton contains. As a result, the quality of the EFAs in these fish is not as high as that of 'free range' fish. Fish which naturally feed on plankton are the oiliest. The plankton in the cold polar oceans is the richest source of EPA and this explains why the Eskimos are so healthy. EPA acts as nature's antifreeze and it allows plankton to survive very cold temperatures. The colder the water, the more EPA is produced by the plankton and this becomes fish fodder.

Cooking Fish

The best way to reap the many benefits of oily fish is to eat the fish raw and if you are a fan of Japanese cuisine, you should enjoy this. For others, the very thought of eating raw fish turns the stomach, although this is the feeling of most people until they have actually tried it. Raw fish has a surprisingly subtle, creamy flavour. To prepare your own raw fish it is important to ensure that it is very, very fresh, preferably killed that day, otherwise you may end up with an upset stomach. Fish oils degrade very quickly which is why old fish smell so terrible. Raw fish can be frozen first to kill any parasites.

If you prefer to cook your fish before eating it, it is best to bake it, as this will preserve the essential fatty acids in the fish more effectively than grilling or frying.

FABULOUS FISH RECIPES

Here are a selection of very different and delicious fish recipes to get you started on the oily fish diet.

Baked fish with pine nut and garlic sauce

(Serves 6)
700–900g (1½–2lb) fillets of oily fish such as mackerel,
    herring, trout or cod
juice of ½ lemon
1tbsp (15ml) olive oil
chopped fresh parsley
salt and pepper
For the sauce
100g (4oz) pine nuts
2 garlic cloves, crushed
2tbsp (30ml) lemon juice
2tbsp (30ml) olive oil
salt and pepper

Place the fish fillets in an oven-proof dish, sprinkle with the lemon juice, olive oil and parsley, and season with salt and pepper. Cover and bake in the oven at 180ºC/350ºF/gas mark 5 for 20–30 minutes or until the fish is cooked through.

Meanwhile, place the pine nuts and garlic in a food processor or blender, season with salt and pepper and process until fairly smooth. Slowly trickle in the lemon juice, then the olive oil, and continue to process until the sauce is thick and creamy. Pour the sauce over the fish and return to the oven to heat through, or reheat in a saucepan and serve as a separate accompaniment.

Fast fish risotto

(Serves 6)
300g (4oz) fresh oily fish
3 onions, peeled and finely chopped
2tbsp (30ml) olive oil
1½ mugs brown rice
450g (15oz) peas
3tbsp freshly chopped basil or parsley

Cook the fish under a hot grill for about 5 minutes, turning it once. Allow to cool slightly, then flake the flesh into large pieces. Heat the oil in a large frying pan and lightly fry the onion. Add the fish, the rice and peas. Stir continuously to prevent the mixture sticking to the sides of the saucepan. Heat for 4–5 minutes to cook the peas. Garnish with the chopped basil or parsley before serving.

Seafood spears

(Serves 4)
For the marinade
4tbsp (60ml) unrefined sunflower or safflower oil
juice of one lemon
1tbsp (15ml) tamari sauce
1tbsp (15ml) fresh chopped parsley
freshly ground black pepper
For the spears
8 shallots, peeled, or 2 large onions, peeled and quartered
750g (1½lb) fresh salmon or tuna

8 scallops or large prawns
1/2 red pepper and 1/2 green pepper, de-seeded and cubed
2 courgettes, thickly sliced
For the garnish
1tbsp chopped fresh parsley

Combine the ingredients for the marinade. Blanch the shallots or onions for 1 minute in boiling water. Cut the fish into chunks and thread together with the scallops or prawns, shallots or onions, pepper and courgettes on to wooden or metal skewers. Brush with the marinade and place under a medium grill and cook for about five minutes (depending upon the fish). Turn the kebabs twice, brushing them with the marinade as they cook. Garnish with chopped parsley before serving.

Gourmet chickpea and tuna salad

(Serves 4–6)
400g (14oz) dried chickpeas soaked overnight in cold water,
*   or 2x400g (14oz) can chickpeas, drained and rinsed*
5tbsp (75ml) olive oil
1 onion, roughly chopped
1 bay leaf
2 garlic cloves
For the tuna
3tbsp (45ml) olive oil
225g (8oz) fresh tuna, cut into chunks
2tbsp (30ml) dry sherry or Japanese mirin flavouring
For the salad dressing
6tbsp (60ml) olive oil
2tbsp lemon juice
2 large tomatoes, skinned and chopped
3 small red onions, finely diced
50g (2oz) pitted black olives
50g (2oz) pitted green olives
salt and pepper

Drain the dried chickpeas, put them in a large saucepan, cover with fresh water and bring to the boil. Boil rapidly for 15 minutes, then transfer the chickpeas to a deep casserole and add the olive oil, onion, bay leaf and whole, skinned garlic cloves. (The canned chickpeas can be used at once.) Add enough water to cover the chickpeas by about 1cm (½inch) and bake in the oven at 120ºC/250ºF/gas mark 1–2 for at least six hours or overnight. In the morning, remove the chopped onion, bay leaf and garlic and the chickpeas are ready to use.

To make the salad dressing, mix the olive oil with the lemon juice and tomatoes and stir in the olives and onions.

To cook the tuna, heat the olive oil in a frying pan or wok, add the tuna and fry quickly until lightly browned. This will take only a very short time, eg 1 minute. Add the sherry or mirin and cook for a further 2–3 minutes. Combine the cooked tuna with the chickpeas and pour the salad dressing over. Mix well and serve warm.

Salmon with Watercress Sauce

(Serves 4)
1 bunch watercress, chopped
1 bunch spring onions, chopped
1 tbsp olive oil
100 ml vegetable stock
100g (4oz) low-fat soft cheese with garlic and herb seasoning
4 salmon fillets

Sauté the chopped onions and watercress in the oil, stirring frequently until softened, add the stock and simmer for five minutes. Liquidize the watercress mixture, add the soft cheese and whizz again if necessary. Meanwhile, grill the salmon skin side up for 2 minutes, turn over and continue to grill for 2-4 minutes depending on the thickness of the fish.

Serve the salmon with the sauce and seasonal vegetables.

Warm Seafood and Pasta Salad

(Serves 4)

2 cloves garlic, crushed
2cm (1in) fresh ginger, grated
1 bunch spring onions, chopped
1 tbsp olive oil
3 tbsp white wine or stock
350g (12oz) mixed seafood, e.g. shrimps, clams, squid etc.
2 tbsp chopped fresh herbs, e.g. dill, coriander, parsley etc.
4 tbsp low-calorie dressing or mayonnaise
275g (10oz) fresh pasta, e.g linguine, tagliatelle
1 lemon or lime

Sauté the garlic, ginger and spring onions in the oil for 2-3 minutes until softened. Add the white wine or stock and allow to bubble for 2 minutes before adding the seafood. Cook for a further 2 minutes to heat through. Remove from the heat and stir in the herbs and low-calorie dressing. Meanwhile, cook the pasta and drain. Serve the pasta topped with the seafood and garnished with lemon or lime wedges.

Fillets of Sole with Pink Grapefruit and Lime

(Serves 4)

Pink grapefruits have a gentle sweetness that complements the richness of the sole prepared here in a not-too-creamy sauce. Fillets of plaice can be used instead of sole.

450g (1lb) fillets of lemon sole, skin removed
salt and cayenne pepper to season
400g (14oz) long grain rice
1 pink grapefruit
350g (12oz) new carrots, scraped
350g (12oz) broccoli, cut into florets
15g (1/2 oz) butter
juice 1/2 lemon
45ml (3fl oz) dry vermouth or white wine

2 tsp cornflour
2 tbsp low fat crème fraîche
Garnish
4 slices lime

To season the fish, combine a pinch of cayenne pepper with 3-4 pinches of fine salt. Sprinkle over the fish then fold the fillets in half so that the whitest side is uppermost and set aside. Put the rice on to cook according to instructions. To segment the grapefruit, remove the top and bottom with a sharp knife, stand on one end, then pare away the skin and pith by cutting down the curved side of the fruit. Remove segments from the grapefruit by working the knife in between the sections. Set aside.

Bring a kettle of water to the boil and put the carrots and broccoli in two separate saucepans, each with a pinch of salt, cover with water and cook both for 6 minutes. Put the butter and lime juice in a large shallow pan. Lay the folded fillets over the top, then pour in the vermouth and 75 ml (3fl oz) water. Bring to a gentle simmer, cover and cook for not more than one minute. Lift the fillets out onto a warm plate. Mix the cornflour with 1 tbsp of cold water, add to the cooking juices, stir and simmer to thicken. Add the crème fraîche, grapefruit segments and season to taste with salt and cayenne pepper. Arrange the fillets onto 4 plates, spoon on the sauce and serve with carrots, broccoli and rice.

Tropical Fish Salad with a Hot Mango Dressing
(Serves 4)

If you were on a dream holiday somewhere hot and tropical, the chances are you would eat nothing but fresh fish, salad and fruit. The chances of taking such a holiday may be slim, but here is an opportunity to indulge in an exotic feast of your own. A fishmonger can prepare the fish to make life easier.

4 black bream, red fish or mullet, scaled and gutted each
     weighing about 275g (10 oz)
2 tbsp olive oil
salt and freshly ground black pepper to season
Mango dressing
1 large ripe mango
1cm (1/2 in) fresh root ginger, peeled and chopped
1/2 tsp chilli paste
2 tbsp lemon or lime juice
3 tbsp freshly chopped coriander leaf
1 batavian, endive or escarole lettuce
75g (3oz) lambs lettuce or corn salad
12 cherrry tomatoes, halved

Pre-heat a moderate grill or light a barbecue and let the embers
settle to a steady glow. Slash the fish deeply on both sides, brush
lightly with oil, season well and set aside. To make the mango
dressing, remove the top and bottom from the flat oval of the
mango, stand on one cut end and pare away the thin skin.
Remove the flesh from both sides of the flat fibrous stone. Slice
one half of the mango flesh for use in the salad later, and put the
remainder in a food processor with the ginger, lime, chilli and
coriander. Process until smooth. Transfer to a serving dish and
set aside. Put the fish on to grill or barbecue for 6-8 minutes
turning once. Wash the salad leaves and dry, then distribute
between four large plates. Place a fish on each and decorate with
slices of mango and tomato.

Mackerel Fillets
   (Serves 4)
   2 large mackerel, filleted
   2 tbsp parmesan cheese, grated
   2 cloves garlic, crushed
   juice and rind of 1 large lemon
   2-3 tbsp chopped fresh parsley

Rinse the mackerel fillets and place skin side down in a large, greased ovenproof dish. In a bowl, mix together the parmesan cheese, garlic, the juice and rind of the lemon and the parsley. Spread the paste over the fillets and cook in the oven or microwave. Serve with new potatoes (if available) and seasonal vegetables.

Salad Nicoise

(Serves 4)

1 crisp lettuce, washed and separated into leaves
225g (8 oz) fresh tuna, cut into chunks
1 tbsp olive oil
8 anchovies
4 free-range eggs (hard boiled)
175g (6 oz) green beans (cooked)
500g (1 lb) ripe tomatoes, sliced
½ cucumber, sliced
1 tbsp fresh parsley, chopped
1 tbsp fresh basil, chopped
2 tbsp (60 ml) simple French dressing (made from 4 parts olive
oil, 1 part white wine vinegar – seasoned with black pepper)

To cook the tuna, heat the olive oil in a frying pan and fry for three to four minutes until cooked through, then allow to cool. Line a bowl or plate with the lettuce leaves and flake the tuna over the centre. Then add half the chopped herbs, the green beans, sliced tomatoes and garnish with the quarters of hard boiled egg, the anchovies and the remaining herbs. Finally, pour over the French dressing.

Glossary

Amino acid – a building block of protein. The body uses over twenty amino acids to form skin, blood, hair, nails and other body tissues.

Antioxidant – a substance that protects cells from damage by free-radicals.

Arachidonic acid – an unsaturated fatty acid made from linoleic acid by enzymes in the body. It has inflammatory properties.

Cholesterol – a fat-like substance that surrounds body cells and is needed to produce hormones, maintain nerve fibres and carry fats and nutrients around the body.

Docosahexaenoic acid (DHA) – one of the two main long-chain omega-3 polyunsaturates found in fish oils.

Double-blind tests – a type of test used by scientists to measure the effectiveness of a new drug, herb or other medicinal substance against an existing remedy or placebo. Neither the participants nor the testers know who is receiving which substance. The identity of those who received the new remedy is only revealed after the results have been recorded. Double-blind testing is an approved and highly effective way of testing the safety and efficacy of new medicines.

Eicosapentaenoic acid (EPA) – one of the two main long-chain omega-3 polyunsaturates found in fish oils.

Essential fatty acids (EFAs) – polyunsaturated and monoun-saturated fats which we must get from food because they cannot be made in the body. They are 'essential' because they are needed for good health.

Free-radical – a reactive compound that is a normal by-product of the body's metabolism, but which can be damaging in high quantities. Air pollution, cigarette smoke and radiation can encourage their formation. Free-radicals react with the fat in cell membranes and change their shape or function.

Hydrogenation – the process of combining polyunsaturated oils with hydrogen to convert them into solid fat. A wide-spread and controversial process over which health questions have recently been raised.

Leukotrienes – hormone-like chemicals with inflammatory properties.

Lipids – fats or oils.

Metabolism – chemical process taking place in living cells which may be divided in to constructive (building-up) or destructive (breaking-down) processes.

Monounsaturated fatty acids – fatty acids which have one double bond. They seem to have a cholesterol-lowering effect on the blood.

Parathyroid – small endocrine glands which control calcium and phosphate metabolism. They are usually found near the thyroid gland.

Polamines – toxic amino acids.

Polyunsaturated fatty acids – fats containing two or more double bonds which reduce cholesterol levels.

Prostaglandins – complex hormone-like chemicals which control biological functions in the body.

Scrofula – tuberculosis of lymph nodes causing the formation of abcesses on the skin.

Synovial fluid – the fluid that lubricates the joints.

Synovial membrane – a joint's protective covering.

Thyroid gland – a ductless gland that lies in front of the trachea. It secretes thyroxine which controls metabolism, growth and development.

Triglyceride – the basic structure of all fats and oils. Also a fatty component in the blood. High levels are related to heart disease.

Ulcerative colitis – inflammation and ulceration of the colon and rectum.

Useful Addresses

Arthritis and Rheumatism Council
Copeman House
St Mary's Court
St Mary's Gate
Chesterfield
Derbyshire S41 7TD
Tel: 01246 558033

British Heart Foundation
14 Fitzhardinge Street
London W1H 4DH
Tel: 0171-935 0185

Fish Foundation
PO Box 24
Tiverton
Devon EX16 4QQ
Tel: 01884 257 547

National Eczema Society
4 Tavistock Place
Tavistock Square
London WC1H 9RA

Psoriasis Association
7 Milton Street
Northampton
Tel: 01604 711129

Seven Seas
Hedon Road
Marfleet
Hull
HU9 5NJ

Index

A

Arthritis 24, 35-44
  case histories 41-4
  osteoarthritis 35-6, 43-4
  rheumatoid 24, 35-6,
    38-41
Asthma/hay fever 62-3

B

Bone/joint disorders 12-13,
  15, 19-21, 31, 37-44, 59,
  63-4
  arthritis 24, 35-44
  osteoporosis 21, 63-4
  rickets 12-13, 15, 19-21, 37

C

Cancer 67-8
Cholesterol 25-9, 71, 83

D

Diet 26, 31-2, 40-1, 48, 51,
  66, 71-81
  for arthritis 40-1
  Eskimo 23, 26, 48, 66, 71
  high-fish/oil-fish 26, 71-81
  Japanese 32, 73
  Mediterranean 71-2
Dosage of cod liver oil 33

E

Early production of cod liver
  oil 14-16
Essential fatty acids (EFAs)
  19, 22-4, 26-7, 40, 46-50,
  52, 54-5, 61, 68-9, 72-3, 84
  DHA 22-3, 26-7, 50, 60-2,
    72
  EPA 22-3, 26-7, 30, 47-50,
    54-5, 68, 72-3
Evening primrose oil 23, 54-6
Exercise 42-3, 64

F

Fish
  choosing the right 69
  cooking 69

H

Heart disease 21, 23, 25-32,
  48, 59, 66-7, 71

I

Immune system 41, 61
Infant formula 57

M

Medicinal properties of cod
  liver oil 11-13, 31-2
  see also specific disorders –
  eg Arthritis, Asthma, etc

Minerals 40-1, 56-7, 63-4
   calcium 40-1, 53, 63-4
   selenium 41
   zinc 56
Multiple sclerosis (MS) 64-5

P
Pregnancy 61-2
Prostaglandins 23, 40, 47-8, 55, 64, 85

R
Recipes 74-81
Rheumatism 11-12, 20
   see also Arthritis, rheumatoid
Rickets 12-13, 15, 19-21, 37

S
Scientific research into cod liver oil 19-33
Skin disorders/skin care 12, 19-20, 31, 45-57, 71
   acne 56-7
   dermatitis 53

   eczema 51-6, 71
   psoriasis 46-51, 71
   scrofula 12, 20
Smoking 28, 65-66

T
Teeth 64
Thrombosis 66-7, 71
Trials 30-31
Triglycerides 28-30

V
Vitamins 12-13, 19-22, 24-5, 40-1, 47-8, 56-7, 62, 64
   A (retinol) 13, 19-21, 24-5, 47-8, 56-7
   B 17
   D 12-13, 19-21, 24-5, 40, 64
   E 21-2, 41, 47, 56-7
   synthetic vitamin pills 20-1

W
Welfare Foods scheme in wartime 16-17

HOW TO ORDER YOUR BOXTREE BOOKS BY LIZ EARLE

Liz Earle's Quick Guides

Available Now

❏ 1 85283 542 7	Aromatherapy	£3.99
❏ 1 85283 544 3	Baby and Toddler Foods	£3.99
❏ 1 85283 543 5	Food Facts	£3.99
❏ 1 85283 546 X	Vegetarian Cookery	£3.99
❏ 0 7522 1619 8	Evening Primrose Oil	£3.99
❏ 0 7533 1614 7	Herbs for Health	£3.99
❏ 1 85283 984 8	Successful Slimming	£3.99
❏ 1 85283 989 9	Vitamins and Minerals	£3.99
❏ 1 85283 979 1	Detox	£3.99
❏ 0 7522 1635 X	Hair Loss	£3.99
❏ 0 7522 1636 8	Youthful Skin	£3.99
❏ 0 7522 1680 5	Healthy Pregnancy	£3.99
❏ 0 7522 1636 8	Dry Skin and Eczema	£3.99
❏ 0 7522 1626 0	Juicing	£3.99
❏ 0 7522 1645 7	Beating Cellulite	£3.99
❏ 0 7522 1673 2	Food Combining	£3.99
❏ 0 7522 1690 2	Post-natal Health	£3.99
❏ 0 7522 1675 9	Food Allergies	£3.99
❏ 0 7522 1685 6	Healthy Menopause	£3.99
❏ 0 7522 1668 6	Beating PMS	£3.99
❏ 0 7522 1663 5	Antioxidants	£3.99

ACE Plan Titles

❏ 1 85283 518 4	Liz Earle's Ace Plan The New Guide to Super Vitamins A, C and E	£4.99
❏ 1 85283 554 0	Liz Earle's Ace Plan Weight-Loss for Life	£4.99

All the books shown opposite are available at your local bookshop or can be ordered direct from the publisher. Just tick the titles you want and fill in the form below. Prices and availability subject to change without notice.

Boxtree Cash Sales,
PO Box 11, Falmouth, Cornwall TR10 9EN

Please send cheque or postal order for the value of the book(s), and add the following for postage and packing:

UK including BFPO – £1.00 for one book, plus 50p for the second book, and 30p for each additional book ordered up to a £3.00 maximum.
Overseas including Eire – £2.00 for the first book, plus £1.00 for the second book, and 50p for each additional book ordered.

OR
please debit this amount from my Access/VISA card (delete as appropriate)

Card number ☐☐☐☐☐☐☐☐☐☐☐☐☐☐☐☐☐☐

Amount £...

Expiry date on card ....

Signed ....

Name ....

Address ....

....

....